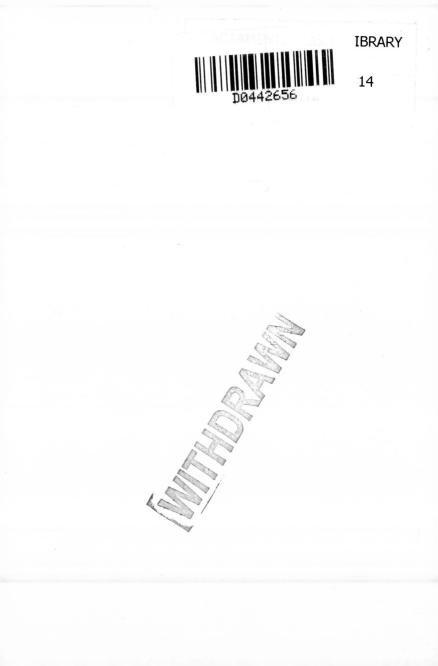

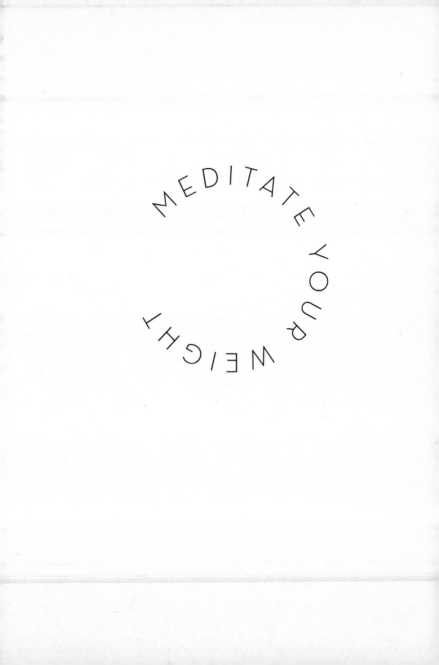

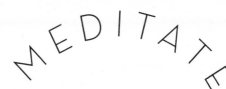

MEDITATE YOUR WEIGHT

A 21-DAY RETREAT TO
OPTIMIZE YOUR METABOLISM
AND FEEL GREAT

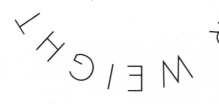

TIFFANY CRUIKSHANK, LAc, MAOM
with MARISKA VAN AALST

HARMONY
BOOKS • NEW YORK

All rights reserved.
Published in the United States by Harmony Books, an imprint
of the Crown Publishing Group, a division of Penguin Random
House LLC, New York.
www.crownpublishing.com

Harmony Books is a registered trademark, and the Circle
colophon is a trademark of Penguin Random House LLC.

Library of Congress Cataloging-in-Publication Data

Cruikshank, Tiffany.
   Meditate your weight : a 21-day retreat to optimize your
metabolism and feel great / Tiffany Cruikshank.
      pages cm
1. Weight loss—Psychological aspects. 2. Metabolism—
Regulation. I. Title.
   RM222.2.C767 2016
   613.2'5—dc23

                        2015033619

ISBN 978-0-8041-8796-1
eBook ISBN 978-0-8041-8797-8

PRINTED IN THE UNITED STATES OF AMERICA

Yoga illustrations by Katie Holeman
Jacket design by Kalena Schoen

10 9 8 7 6 5 4 3 2 1

First Edition

This book is dedicated to every person

who has ever struggled with her

self-worth, her body, or her potential.

May this book help you to cultivate a

healthy body and a nourishing mental

outlook, and to discover your value and

worth, as well as the immense beauty

that lives inside of you.

Contents

MEDITATE YOUR WEIGHT

Introduction

Every day, all day, we are bombarded with messages from social media, family, coworkers, Photoshopped ads telling us that we're not enough—we need to eat healthier, lose weight, look skinnier. It can be virtually impossible not to feel like you *should* look better or you *should* feel better, regardless of who you are.

With all this noise swirling around in our heads, figuring out where these messages stop and where our own best instincts toward health begin can be very difficult. In our struggle with these body-policing messages, we often unconsciously capitulate—or we resist their tyranny by rebelling against healthy changes—and end up hurting ourselves in the process.

We all know that the apple and kale are better for us than the doughnut, but somehow we still end up choosing the doughnut. We all know that going for a walk or to the gym will help us lose weight more than watching TV will, but we still end up on the couch. And even when we choose the apple and the gym, we sometimes still end up hitting a wall when it comes to feeling our best. We'll consult doctors, run tests to check that our thyroid, digestion, reproductive hormones, or adrenal glands are functioning properly—yet we may still not have an answer to our stubborn health woes. We still don't feel good. What's going on here?

I have a theory. I believe that the most powerful ally in the quest for vibrant health is one that's often overlooked: the huge capacity of the mind-body connection.

THE MIND-BODY CONNECTION

The mind-body connection is actually a bit mislabeled. Our "mind" lives in our nervous system, which is most definitely part of the "body." What happens in the mind can create a direct physical effect on the rest of the body. In that way, you can say there really isn't a "connection"—they are one and the same.

And yet we know intuitively that they *are* different. A thought is just a thought—it's not completely automatic, like your heartbeat. Thoughts are more like breaths or the blinks of an eye—these can happen without our awareness but also can be studied and shifted with awareness, even if just temporarily.

When we neglect to pay attention to the mind-body connection, we might do everything "right" and still find ourselves frustrated in our health and weight-loss goals.

As a master yoga teacher, founder of Yoga Medicine, sports medicine expert, and practitioner of Chinese medicine, I have specialized in helping my patients and students optimize their health for more than a decade. And in that time, with thousands of patients and students, I've found, over and over, that ignoring the power of the mind can be the primary limiting factor in our health.

TRAINING THE BRAIN

When highly trained, the brain can help us achieve any goal, no matter what aspect of our lives—from scoring that promotion at work to having a healthy pregnancy and delivery to losing twenty pounds. But often our brain limits us. Sometimes it hampers our ability to follow through. Sometimes it makes us give in to cravings. Sometimes we just plain live up to our own low expectations.

But these very human tendencies don't necessarily mean we need to rush that brain to the psychiatrist. In fact, many of us share the exact same types of self-limiting thought patterns. And because these patterns are so universal, we have decades, even millennia, of great experience in what works to help change them.

In meditation, the goal is not so much to eliminate these thinking patterns as it is to identify them. Once we get clear about what's happening inside our head and how it affects the rest of our functioning, it's easier for our brain to make decisions that align with our true health goals. Recognizing unhelpful thought patterns allows us to directly address them through the use of simple meditations and mental af-

firmations (mantras) that help us achieve our goals—
such as to lose weight.

Decades of medical research have shown us that
meditation is powerful medicine. Studies have proven
that meditation does the following:

- reduces heart rate and blood pressure
- reduces stress hormones
- reduces pain and inflammation
- reduces depression and anxiety
- improves immune system function
- improves focus and memory
- improves a sense of peaceful calm
- improves the feeling of connectedness
- improves sleep

That's just the tip of the iceberg. The research on meditation's power continues to grow more compelling—
and one of the promising lines of research concerns
meditation's effect on our weight-loss efforts. For example, multiple studies have found that meditation
helps improve our awareness of internal hunger and
satiety signals, as well as our ability to regulate what
and how much we eat.[1] Meditation has been shown
to reduce cravings for unhealthy food[2] and decrease
the frequency of binge eating and emotional eating.[3]

Meditation can also reduce high levels of the stress hormone cortisol and resulting toxic belly fat.[4] One study even found that an eight-week meditation class tripled the amount of weight lost by a group of elderly women, when compared with those who did not use similar techniques.[5]

Of course, meditation is not a magic wand—we still have to nourish ourselves with healthy foods and exercise. But meditation is an incredible supplement to *any* kind of weight-loss regimen, creating a multiplying effect on your preferred approach. When you make the commitment to try even five minutes of meditation a day, you strengthen and train your mind to more easily support your goals and your metabolism.

And then anything is possible.

THE MEDITATE YOUR WEIGHT PROGRAM

Over the course of my decades of work with patients and students, I've identified some very common self-limiting thought patterns and developed meditations to help draw awareness to those patterns. I've given a lot of thought to selecting the meditations, reflections, and mantras included in this book, choosing only those that I've found most effective for resetting the metabolic engine.

The 21-day program in this book is a structured, progressive, mind-training sequence. All of the meditations and exercises help you first identify and then address the thought patterns that are holding you back from achieving your health and wellness goals. Just as any athlete follows her coach's program to help her train for a race or competition, you can follow this program to help you train your mind for optimal health and wellness. To live with more energy, feel stronger and leaner, look radiant, and reach the best possible state of health doesn't mean starving ourselves or running a marathon—but it does require us to live with greater awareness.

Part 1 is a crash course in the miracle of meditation—how it works and how it can benefit every part of your body and your mind. In the first three chapters we'll delve into the science—exactly *why* is meditation so effective in helping us attain our goals? I'll also share details about my own experience with patients and yoga students, and how I've used these methods to help them, and myself, to heal.

In chapter 1 I'll explain the basics of meditation

and address some common misconceptions about it. In chapter 2 we'll uncover exactly which stumbling blocks—both physical and mental—may be impeding your weight loss, and how meditation can help you get past them. In chapter 3 we'll dig a little deeper to learn how meditation can change your physiology on a cellular, even genetic, level. You'll discover how meditation has been scientifically proven to physically alter the shape, size, and functioning of your brain, to chemically alter the endocrine system, and to tone and soothe the nervous and cardiovascular systems. You'll see exactly how meditation reroutes self-defeating neural patterns that can keep you stuck, and how these brain-based changes can help set your body up for weight loss success.

Once you understand my background, my approach, and the scientific research behind the effectiveness of meditation, you'll start to see how just five or ten or twenty minutes, once a day, can lead to radical changes in your health and happiness.

In part 2 we begin the 21-day retreat. Each day I'll introduce you to a specific theme that I have found integral to metabolic success. I'll share my personal experiences with this topic, or a patient story, some interesting facts or cutting-edge research. And throughout the 21 days I will also share the ways in which meditation can deepen your engagement with life and your awareness of the wonder and beauty all around you. Life will get lighter, which may be even more important than any weight loss goal you have.

From there you'll enter your daily meditation—just three minutes to start, adding on time as you feel ready. I'll talk you through all the basics—how to sit, where to sit, what you'll use to sit, and more—as well as provide a mental image, idea, or phrase to guide you. Directly after, I ask you to respond to two or three short journal prompts, to help you investigate and reflect upon how each theme reveals itself in your life. Finally, I'll send you on your way with your daily mantra and some intentions for the day, asking you to pay attention to thoughts, emotions, sensations, and experiences to help you consider and reflect upon the topic at hand.

The next day's lesson will build on the prior day's lesson and deepen your self-awareness as you develop a daily practice. Each day of the program will follow the same format, so you can more easily settle into a rhythm. My hope is that by the end of the 21 days you'll have made your meditation practice a simple habit that's easy to keep integrated into your already very full life.

Whether you've wanted to meditate your whole

life and haven't found the right format or you're a seasoned meditator who wants to expand your practice to optimize your metabolism, I hope you find what you need in this book. My goal is to show you just how simple and practical the tool of meditation really is, and how incredibly powerful your results can be, all in just a few minutes a day.

Most of all, I hope you find the next three weeks to be an enjoyable lesson in YOU—what makes you tick, what holds you back, what makes you come alive, and how you can help yourself be fully present, with your arms and eyes wide open, in all areas of your life.

Let's get started!

WHAT'S WEIGHING YOU DOWN?

Part 1

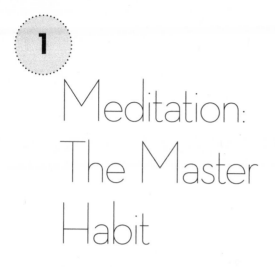

1

Meditation: The Master Habit

I will never forget working with Leslie.

Leslie was very disciplined and worked extremely hard to lose weight. She followed a clean diet. She worked out at the gym regularly. But no matter what she did, she could not get her body to let go of those last fifteen pounds she wanted to lose to feel healthy again. She'd been successful at reducing her weight in the past. But this time, no luck.

When Leslie came to my office and shared her current program with me, I was struck by all the work she'd done to lose weight. There really weren't any additional diet- or exercise-related changes she could make—she'd been *that* disciplined. She was even aware that working out too hard or eating too little could stimulate counterproductive stress hormones, so she'd also been focused on striking a healthy balance between the two and on reducing stress in other areas of her life.

Leslie had done everything that I would have recommended, with the exception of one critical ingredient for success: She had not yet started to meditate.

When I suggested she begin meditation, she was skeptical but game. "I've always wanted to try meditation," she said. "Even if I don't lose weight, maybe this program will help me stick with it."

Leslie started with five minutes a day, working up to ten minutes once she felt ready. Initially, she struggled to find the time in her busy schedule, but then she quickly came to see meditation as a highlight of her day. And sure enough, shortly after coming to see me—making no other changes to her self-care routine—Leslie had lost fifteen pounds. I continued to see her once or twice a year for a few years, and she has maintained that loss, seemingly effortlessly—looking more serene (and younger!) each time I see her.

I've watched many men and women spend a tremendous amount of time perfecting their diet and exercise regimes—really pushing themselves toward clean diets, yoga, high-performance athletics, and more—but remaining frustrated and unhappy with their results. Some struggle with consistency, battling inner demons they can't seem to defeat, and get pulled back into self-sabotaging habits. Others, like Leslie, can motivate themselves to do all the right things, but they still don't see the changes they want, and they don't feel their best. Patients often come to me in tears, wondering what else they could possibly do to break through this frustrating plateau. Many have done everything possible to tell their bodies that they want to be at a different weight. But just like Leslie, they need to make the final, critical connection: They need to relay that message to their minds.

Leslie was still operating with outdated ideas about herself. In her mind she was an overweight woman. She hadn't yet started to visualize herself at her target weight—and her fixed image of herself ensured that her body would hold on to those fifteen pounds, no matter what. Her brain—the master of her nervous system, the captain of the whole body—needed to believe the change was possible in order to allow the biochemical changes necessary to make it happen.

Meditation changed her perspective and helped her have faith in her image of herself as lean and vital. Her daily meditation practice and the resulting mental shift was all it took for her body to let go of those last fifteen pounds.

Whether I'm working with stressed-out college students or hard-charging executives, new moms or recent retirees, I have seen that meditation can be a very simple but transformative solution to all manner of stubborn and frustrating problems. In our quest for more vibrant health and happiness, many of us are held back by subconscious messages and long-standing patterns. We might not even know our blocks exist, even as we run headlong into them, day after day. But as little as five minutes of mindful meditation, practiced daily, can help us become aware of our blocks—which is often the first and most important step to getting past them.

As meditation helps you see your blocks, you begin to understand the connection between the hidden messages you're sending to yourself, the self-defeating patterns you unconsciously follow, and the frustrating lack of progress you've made toward your goals. But rather than nudging you into a self-chastising spiral, meditation helps you develop greater understanding of and compassion for yourself, foibles and all. It is in this space of peace and self-compassion that your body relaxes its defenses, opens up, and reveals its innate instinct for health—often enabling natural, automatic, even effortless weight loss.

As we make meditation a regular part of our daily lives, we experience small "aha!" moments that progress to ever-richer insights. These changes start to compound as we become stronger and less engaged with our fears. We develop the courage to turn and face the biggest problems in our lives, painful issues we may have avoided facing for years—issues that often turn out to be the very root causes of some of our most frustrating blocks.

These foundational shifts may take a while to occur, but once we address them, life suddenly seems easier, richer, more meaningful. We begin to heal lifelong injuries, reboot long-dormant dreams, and set off on paths that had previously seemed inaccessible.

And all of this begins with just a few minutes

a day. When you tap the power of meditation, your quest to remove extra pounds is often just the beginning of a truly life-changing transformation.

SIMPLE BUT MIGHTY

The practice of meditation is actually very simple: You require nothing but an intention to quiet your mind for a few moments. You don't need any equipment or extensive training—you don't even necessarily need a quiet space (although it is handy). As simple as meditation is, its powerful effects have been studied and validated by the most prestigious medical institutions in the world. Millions of people have been subjected to sleep studies, blood tests, brain scans, and all manner of clinical trials to chronicle its effects on our various body systems. This research has proven that meditation has a verifiable, physical effect on how our bodies manage stress; it changes our physiology, our nervous and endocrine systems, even the very structure of our brains.

Meditation can support almost any effort to improve health—including the pursuit of a healthy weight. In fact, a recent analysis of peer-reviewed studies that looked at mindfulness-based interventions to address eating behaviors related to weight gain—including overeating, binge eating, and emotional eating—found that participants in 86 percent of the mindfulness studies demonstrated improvement in their weight-related goals.[1]

Research shows that meditation, and especially mindfulness meditation, aids weight loss efforts in the following ways:

- by teaching us to slow down and truly savor our food, so we enjoy it more and need less to feel satisfied
- by helping us understand what actual physical hunger and fullness feel like, instead of eating out of habit or craving
- by helping us question those cravings that seem "irresistible"

Many studies have shown that mindfulness techniques can reduce food cravings and enhance weight loss. But more awareness can also help us clearly see how our mental habits affect us: Why do we crave certain foods, whether healthy or unhealthy? Why do we have self-limiting mental patterns—and how do those patterns impact our body image, our health, our posture? How do we treat ourselves—and how do we interact with and treat others? How do we feel and live and breathe and move in our lives? All of these questions play a role in our health and our happiness, our level of connection with others and contentment with our lives. If we can start to get at the answers to those questions, the weight loss often comes naturally.

Seem too good to be true? How can simply sitting quietly have that much impact? Maybe you have your doubts about meditation—or you've tried it, but it doesn't seem to work for you. Let's look at a few of the most common myths about meditation to see if we can address those doubts and reservations.

SOME MYTHS ABOUT MEDITATION—AND THE TRUTH

Though meditating is simpler to do than many believe, it is also a mysterious process—how does it work, exactly? Even scientists are not exactly sure, but they're getting closer. That mystery sometimes causes a bit of a PR problem for meditation, but I'd love to clear up a few of those misunderstandings.

Myth:

"MEDITATION IS A SPIRITUAL PRACTICE."

Truth:

**MEDITATION IS, FIRST AND FOREMOST,
A MENTAL PRACTICE.**

Meditation is not voodoo. Meditation is not New Age or mystical. Yes, meditation *has* been used in many forms in religious traditions and cultures throughout history and throughout the world—but the act of meditating isn't inherently spiritual.

At its core, meditation is a means of training your mind. It has direct physiological effects on the brain and nervous system that can be studied in the lab, tracked by sophisticated fMRI brain scanners, or analyzed with a blood test, stethoscope, or heart rate monitor. In fact, over the last twenty-five years, more than three thousand studies on meditators have been conducted at some of the most respected research institutions in the world, including Harvard, Yale, Stanford, and the universities of California, North Carolina, and Wisconsin, among many others. The data from these studies is very clear: Meditation helps people lead healthier, happier, and more fulfilling lives.

Myth:

"MEDITATION JUST DOESN'T WORK FOR ME."
OR: "I CAN'T MEDITATE."

Truth:

MEDITATION WORKS FOR EVERYONE,
AND EVERYONE CAN DO IT.

I hear it all the time: "I can't meditate—it just doesn't work for me."

Imagine if a baby who was just learning how to walk tried to take a step and fell down, then turned around and said, "Sorry, Mom and Dad—this walking thing just doesn't work for me."

Silly, right? But meditation is like walking—it's an activity we learn to do in very short spurts, then continue to practice and improve upon for the rest of our lives.

Once you've mastered the basics of walking, you can go in any direction you'd like—you can run the fifty-yard dash in gym class, you can train for a 5k, you can become a marathoner. Or, like many people, you might just stick with basic walking to get you through your days. But the core mechanics involved in each of these activities is exactly the same: You put one foot in front of the other, and you move forward.

Meditation is just like that. You might just do three minutes a day; you might work up to twenty. You might fall in love with it and decide to dig deep and do a retreat. But at an elemental level, no matter where you find yourself currently, you are a meditator. From the very first moment you sit, take a breath, and notice that your mind is wandering, you're already doing it—you're meditating.

Myth:

"THE *REAL* TYPE OF MEDITATION IS [X]—AND IF YOU DON'T DO [X], YOU'RE NOT *REALLY* MEDITATING."

Truth:

**ANY TYPE OF MEDITATION IS "REAL";
NO ONE TYPE IS BETTER THAN ANOTHER.**

When we start meditating, a common trap is to get caught in thinking we have to follow a specific type of meditation. When I first got into meditation back in the early nineties, people were very specific about it. I heard all kinds of dictums:

- You can't be sitting on a chair—you have to sit on a cushion.
- Your legs need to be in this position.

- You have to have your right thumb on top and your left thumb on the bottom.
- Your right heel must be in front.
- Your spine has to be right over your pelvis.
- You have to chant this or think about that.

All of these *might* be helpful suggestions to you—or not. To use meditation to reach your health goals, there are truly no absolutes of this kind. What works for you is what works for *you*. It doesn't matter if you do a visualization, or count your breaths, or simply take a moment to close your eyes and be still while riding on the bus—all of these are just tools, and all of them are forms of meditation. Anytime you take a moment to just sit there—voilà, you're meditating.

And that's the ultimate goal of meditation: that, with practice, you will get to a level of comfort in which you can just tip back into that same relaxed, focused mental space on the drop of a dime, anytime you notice that you're getting stressed. By developing your meditation skills, you become able to step out of the stress loop and remain cool, calm, and collected as often as you'd like.

If you're drawn to one specific method of meditation, that's great—stick with what works for you.

Find the tool that you need and use it. But from a scientific perspective, and for the results we're looking for in the mind and body, please know there are many "right" ways to do it.

Myth:
"YOU HAVE TO MEDITATE FOR TWENTY MINUTES OR MORE, OR IT'S NOT WORTH IT."

Truth:
ANY AMOUNT OF MEDITATION CAN MAKE A DIFFERENCE IN YOUR LIFE.

The length of time you spend meditating is absolutely secondary to frequency. If you have to struggle and force yourself to stay still for twenty minutes, you're not going to get the health benefits that you would get from simply sitting for five minutes and just paying attention to your breath. The effort you expend to sit in that spot longer than your tolerance can take will stimulate a stress response in your nervous system. I would so much rather you meditate once a day for three minutes than once a week for twenty.

Yes, that little time really does make a difference. One study found that as few as five minutes of meditation a day for four weeks significantly reduced participants' measures of stress and anxiety and increased their perceived quality of life.[2] Another study found that fifteen minutes of meditation a day reduced participants' measures of stress by up to 36 percent.[3] But even something as simple as a singular, mindful exhale can lower your blood pressure, at least for a moment or two.

Not only does meditation not take a lot of time to be effective, a new line of research suggests that meditation actually changes our *perception* of time—making us feel as though we have *more* of it in our daily lives. Remember in childhood, when the summer felt like it lasted forever? As adults, we lose this sense of luxuriously expansive time. But one German study found that seasoned mindfulness meditators experienced less subjective time pressure, a greater sense of time "expanding," and a general slowing in their experience of the passage of time.[4] Compared with non-meditators, they were more likely to say that the previous week and the previous month had passed "slowly."

Imagine—just a few minutes spent meditating can deepen and expand your experience of time itself. You will have fewer of those "Where did the day go?" moments. Your weekends and vacations will feel longer. You will gain a richness in your moment-to-moment existence that you may not even realize you're not experiencing right now.

Meditation can help you live longer, both in calendar years and in your own subjective experience of those years.

Myth:
"MEDITATION SHOULD BE DIFFICULT—AND IF IT'S NOT DIFFICULT, YOU'RE NOT DOING IT RIGHT."

OR: "MEDITATION SHOULD BE EASY—AND IF IT'S NOT EASY, YOU'RE NOT DOING IT RIGHT."

Truth:
MEDITATION IS SIMPLE—NOT EASY, NOT DIFFICULT. ALLOWING OURSELVES TO EXPERIENCE IT WITHOUT JUDGMENT IS THE TRICK.

People have this idea that meditation has to be difficult to have any impact on their lives. Others believe it has to be easy—as in, "I must be able to do it immediately without any challenge whatsoever, or it's not for me."

Neither one of these is true. But these myths come from the same place: judgment. Meditation helps us recognize that these beliefs are simply thoughts, judgments that our minds have created—not absolute truths that should guide our choice of whether or not to meditate.

Myth:

"IF YOUR MIND WANDERS, YOU'RE NOT A MEDITATOR."

Truth:

NO MIND IS STILL ALL THE TIME.

A lot of people come to the practice with the idea that meditation is about making your mind really still. But just sitting and noticing that your mind is wandering *is* meditation. Even trained monks experience moments when their minds wander off. That never stops.

When our mind wanders, we can start to judge ourselves: *Am I doing it right? Am I doing it wrong? Am I doing it well? Am I doing it poorly?* We get upset with ourselves for it wandering off with all these distractions. But keeping your mind focused on one point is really difficult—in fact, it's almost impossible.

The truth is, your mind is always going to meander—and that wandering *is part of meditation.* The process of repeatedly bringing your mind back, and not scolding it for having taken a detour, *is* meditation. In the mental gym that is meditation, the act of noticing the wandering *is* that biceps curl that will strengthen your brain. You're becoming an observer, rather than a judge—the essential shift that forms the basis of all meditation.

Myth:

"BO-RING! I HAVE NO NEED TO LEARN HOW TO FOCUS—MY BRAIN LOVES MULTITASKING!"

Truth:

NO BRAIN *REALLY* LOVES MULTITASKING.

According to the Laboratory of Neuro Imaging at the University of Southern California, about seventy thousand thoughts travel through our minds on a daily basis.[5] Some of them have to do with swearing after stubbing a toe, or feeling the temperature of the water before we step into the shower, or any other quotidian detail. And some thoughts are biggies—work problems, money concerns, too-much-to-do-in-too-little-time anxieties, painful heartbreak. As intelligent beings, our brains can get easily tempted by all those juicy thoughts. But for most of us, being distracted from the here and now not only exhausts us, it also causes our productivity and happiness to plummet.

One Harvard study used an iPhone app to track how often people's minds wander and how those wanderings affect their level of happiness. They found that no matter what people were doing, from working to shopping to playing with their kids to hanging out with friends, they were much happier when their minds were not wandering. (Note: "Making love" was the activity that showed the *least* amount of mind wandering.) The researchers found that the nature of what people were doing had less impact on their happiness than their degree of mind wandering while doing it. An even deeper analysis of the data suggested that "mind wandering was the cause, not merely the consequence, of their unhappiness."[6]

So why does mind wandering make us unhappy? Part of the answer must be that we lose our sense of flow, that total absorption in our tasks, that research has proven is a potent source of happiness. But unless we are consciously observing all of those mind-wandering thoughts, we may also be experiencing thousands of *judgments* along with them. Meditation helps us be able to sit and watch that judgment, just notice it, without having to make it go away or make it different. If we can resist judgment, we can better manage our nervous system reactivity. Every distracted thought and negative judgment is no longer an opportunity for our fight-or-flight reaction to be triggered and our stress hormone cascade to begin—we can learn how to consciously sidestep the whole business.

Thanks, brain, but I don't want to dance right now—I'm just observing.

THE FOUNDATION OF ALL MEDITATION

Now that we've covered the most common myths about meditation, let's talk a bit more about two core truths that I've alluded to previously. Two concepts or mind-sets form the foundation of all meditation: becoming an observer and practicing non-judgment.

Becoming an Observer

Do you know that feeling of road hypnosis, when you can drive for ten miles without even realizing it? How many times have you driven to work on auto-pilot, reflexively taking the same turns, waiting at the same stoplights, and not noticed the trees or flowers or signs or even the people that you drove by?

Most of us experience this daily. Our gaze becomes fixed; our eyes are open but we are not really seeing. The brain hovers between being marginally alert and actually noticing what's happening around us in this moment. We can float in and out of this haze, off and on for minutes or hours, without really registering the passage of time.

Certainly our nervous system needs to tune out *some* of that detail—if we zeroed in on every passing billboard or pebble on the road, we'd be overwhelmed with minutiae in minutes. But that daydreaming, sleepwalking haze is very different from the sensation of being alertly aware of the space in the mind— the sensation we can develop through meditation practice.

As we spend more time in the state of being present in meditation, we start to notice more things throughout the day, those little details of beauty or quiet majesty that add texture to our lives. Gradually, or even suddenly, we'll start to notice flowers blooming or plants that we'd never taken in before. After just a short period of a sustained meditation practice, our moments start to gain more depth and richness, more sensory detail. And as we notice those things, we'll be better able to catch ourselves when we dip into that "zone-out" state, where we're just going through the motions and not really being present.

Sounds easy, doesn't it? But becoming an observer, watching your thoughts without becoming engaged with them, is probably the hardest part of the meditation practice. Human nature tends to dictate that when we notice something, we automatically dig in—we want to get *involved*.

This common scenario is easily imagined with children. Many parents find that just standing back and watching your kids navigate life without interfering can require a Herculean effort in self-control. We feel the urge to tie the shoelace, to mop up the spill, to correct the mistake on the math homework. Even to give advice. We hear or see an issue, and we want to resolve, to guide, to *rescue*.

Our minds react to our thoughts just like a parent reacts to her child—the mind naturally wants to get involved, to dig in and get to work. This tendency comes from a good place—you just want to help your brain "solve" the issue that's plaguing it. But just as a child's "problem" can often resolve itself without our intervention, we can help our stress level and our well-being by strengthening our resolve to simply watch our thoughts and not get involved.

Our natural inclination to "fix" often shows up during our very first meditation session, when we start to pay attention to the breath. (Note: I'm not talking about specific yoga and meditation practices, such as *pranayama,* in which we actually look at and consciously regulate the breath—those involve a very different approach.) The instructor might begin the meditation session saying something like "Pay attention to your breath"—and your very first thought is, "I'm not breathing the right way!"

In truth, maybe you come to your mat or cushion with your breath choppy or shallow; maybe you're trying to extend your exhale for that "perfect" breath. But as you learn meditation, you'll start to realize that, rather than lengthening, deepening, slowing, or otherwise changing the breath, meditation is about simply *watching* the breath—which is much harder. Your task is not to judge the quality of your breath but to sit there without even subtly trying to modify it in any way—this is great practice in becoming an observer.

Becoming an observer is a skill that helps us in many areas of our lives. Imagine being able to keep a cool head in moments of high stress. You could choose not to escalate an argument with your child or partner. You would be able to see a clear solution in a moment of crisis at work. Becoming an observer also helps us stay aware of what our body is asking for from moment to moment. Then, we can focus on the signals our body is sending us instead of succumbing to the mindless reactivity that can lead to poor food choices.

Training for Non-judgment

Meditation has an amazing way of making every-thing more conscious. Once we start to develop this skill of being an observer, we tune in to the details all around us that we might have been missing when we were simply zombie-walking through our days.

We can use meditation to train the mind in the same way we can use time in the gym to train the body. When we go to the gym, we lift weights to make our biceps stronger and better able to lift things. When we sit in meditation, we train the muscles of the mind to be less reactive and less judgmental.

Why is being nonjudgmental so important, any-way? After all, everyone makes assumptions and judgments about the world around us—that's just a part of being human, isn't it?

Not necessarily. These mental habits we've learned may *feel* like a natural part of being human, but they're not always healthy for us. Yet we fall into them every day. The friend who doesn't return the text or e-mail—she must be mad at you! The photo of a party posted on Facebook—why weren't you invited? The smirk you thought you saw on the barista's face—well, she can forget that tip! The freckle on your face that's changing shape—could it be cancer?

These quick, automatic, unexamined assumptions are not simply innocent or inert—they leave a residue. Our reactions to them have an impact on our brain chemistry, hormonal reactions, cardiac health, inflammation levels—not to mention our general worldview and level of happiness. Unexamined judgments have the potential to change our anxiety level, our moods, even our relationships. If we allow them to, these judgments can define who we are. We need to be able to stop and carefully examine them, and consciously consider whether or not we want to take them in, give them any credence, or offer them residence in our brain.

The better we get at being observers, the more likely we are to notice our judgments. Once our brain starts to notice, we can decide: *Do I want to keep doing that? Is that a rational assumption? Am I as healthy as I want to be? Do I have the energy I'd like? Am I a hard worker? Am I ready to live a cleaner life?* We can start to reorient some of those subconscious thought processes and make them more conscious.

Ultimately, the judgments we have about the world around us are the same as those we have about ourselves—they're thoughts, mental shortcuts, but not reality. Heaping judgment on ourselves, especially about our weight, can be extremely damaging to our health and our self-image. Contrary to all those shaming messages we may have picked up in our youth or from the media, we cannot criticize ourselves into losing weight. Research shows that people who feel a sense of shame about their weight are actually less likely to achieve their health or weight loss goals.

Meditation can help us become aware of these thought habits and learn how to look at them without judgment, so we can eventually help shift them. Becoming an observer and adopting a nonjudgmental stance are the two essential first steps toward approaching our personal blocks with self-compassion and kindness.

In the next chapter we'll talk about what the most common blocks are—and how meditation can help us surmount them.

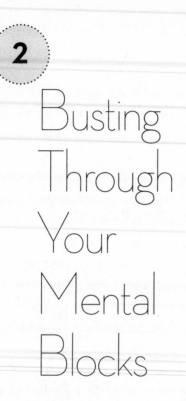

2

Busting Through Your Mental Blocks

Regardless of where you are in your health journey, whenever you try to make a change, you can run up against a big barrier standing in your way: your habits. Science has determined that about 70 percent of

our health and longevity is dictated by our lifestyle—
which is really nothing more than a collection of our
long-term habits.

Most of us have at least one habit we'd prefer to
kick to the curb. But while it can be tempting to go
cold turkey, all-or-nothing attempts to quit bad habits can backfire, causing rebound, self-criticism, and
discouragement. Despite our good intentions, sometimes our brains cling to our habits like security blan-
kets, even when they don't serve us well.

Rather than try to kick it outright, an easier way
to get rid of a habit you don't want is to develop a better one—and allow that good one to gently nudge the
unhelpful one out of the picture. Meditation, in many
ways, is the queen of all good habits. That daily ten
minutes (or five, or even three!) spent in meditation
exerts a tremendous influence over the remaining
twenty-three hours and fifty minutes, totally out of
proportion to the little time required to do it. When
you first focus on developing a meditation practice,
you'll find it's much easier to develop other great
habits—and loosen the grip of unhealthy ones.

I see this phenomenon every day in my practice.
Few more clearly exemplify it than my patient Abby.

A BRIDGE TO NEW HABITS

Abby came to me for treatment when she was having trouble getting pregnant. She'd been trying to conceive for two years, but something wasn't working. Every time she came to my office, she would walk in and set her gigantic thirty-two-ounce soda on my desk. And there it would sit, looming over our entire consultation.

I tried everything I could to get her to stop. I would bring her handouts on why soda was bad for her. I would explain about the connection between sugar and infertility. Even her desire for a child couldn't dissuade her from this habit. No amount of information or research seemed capable of loosening Abby's grip on that soda cup.

Finally I switched gears. We started talking about what the connection was—why did she feel like she needed it? What was she getting from soda? She said she originally started drinking it to give her enough energy to get through the day. And now she'd become so dependent on it, she truly believed it was all that kept her functioning. She was petrified of attempting to navigate her busy life without it.

That huge cup had become her moral support

and her friend, an indispensable companion and ally through her long days. Once we'd clarified the role that soda was playing in her life, it was clear that no amount of discussion about its health risks was going to displace this emotional connection. Instead, we needed to address the *function* of the soda; we needed to find another way to help her feel supported, and we needed to manage her anxiety about not having the energy to get things done.

Her schedule was so packed, she could commit to only three minutes of meditation per day to start, then five minutes per day a week later—but that's really all it took for her to start to recognize her energy patterns and how she could better manage her stress. She cut down a tiny bit, day by day, and slowly but surely, she began to let go of the soda—as well as her concerns about her energy level. To her great surprise, she was still managing her responsibilities quite well. In fact, she seemed to be doing even better without it.

Just weeks later, Abby felt a lot better (and looked great, too). After a little longer, she had lost some weight, but that was just a happy side benefit. The real gift came three months after starting meditation and phasing out soda: After more than two years of trying to conceive and many different procedures (conventional and alternative), Abby got pregnant.

I don't believe she would have seen this wonderful outcome without meditation. Abby's mindfulness program was what allowed her to take a good, close look at her energy level, her nourishment, and exactly what she was getting out of her "relationship" with her daily soda. The time spent in meditation helped her realize she needed to find other solutions for her anxiety—and that she also needed to form closer, more supportive relationships with her colleagues and friends, instead of relying on an extremely unhealthy beverage for moral support.

In my practice I've seen this scenario repeated over and over, with people who are trying to lose weight holding on to patterns and habits that no longer serve them. No matter where we are on our health journey, we may have long-standing emotional connections with our bad habits that make it hard to let them go. Whether our unhelpful habit is sugar or potato chips (or both), or sitting on the couch and not wanting to exercise, or slavishly counting calories and overexercising for hours a day—all of these destructive habits fulfill some need within us. Meditation helps us observe our patterns without judgment, so we can start to learn from them instead of hide from them. Facing these truths helps us get to the bottom of our authentic needs, allowing us to find more empowering, productive, and healthy ways to meet them.

UNRAVELING OUR DESTRUCTIVE HABITS

Health and fitness advice comes at us from all directions. This tsunami of musts, the constant drumbeats of "do this, don't do that," makes us feel like we can never do or be enough. Sometimes the resulting state of being overwhelmed can lead to self-defeating thoughts: *There must be something wrong with me. Everyone else can [avoid sugar/eat vegan/run five miles every day]. Why can't I? If I can't do it right, why even try?*

This all-or-nothing thinking is a mental habit that often gets in our way. But despite our culture's perennial search for silver-bullet solutions, there isn't one and there never will be. Your quest to shed weight is just that: *your* quest. What works for others might not work for you—and nothing works for everyone.

Here's what we know does work: developing compassion for yourself; learning how to sink into the experience of the current moment; and trying not to judge yourself too harshly. Meditation can help you develop all of these beneficial mental habits, training you to stay rooted in the present instead of getting lost in regrets about the past or fears about the future.

As these habits strengthen, they'll start to nudge out less helpful ones, and you can more easily move forward with your health goals. Let's consider some of the unhelpful habits that can pack on pounds, and how meditation can help you address them.

Meditation helps you tune in to your hunger (and other body signals).

A healthy lifestyle and metabolism start with being able to hear your own internal signals. All the messages from your body and your mind can either create stumbling blocks or help you break through them— and they are far easier to hear when you meditate.

Meditation allows you to key in to the biological feedback that tells you how your plan is working: *How does drinking more water change my skin and my appetite? Do those supplements help soothe my joint pain? If I work out in the morning, how does the rest of my day feel?*

One of the most important of these signals is hunger. In all the rush-rush-rush of our lives, sometimes we eat out of habit rather than genuine hunger. We might eat everything on the plate without stopping to check in and see if we really need those last few bites. Or maybe we're just mindlessly following the "Clean your plate!" conditioning we learned as kids.

We may have forgotten what the rumble of true hunger in our belly feels like, or the satisfaction of a meal that leaves us pleasantly full but not stuffed. Instead, what, when, and how much we eat might be determined entirely by external signals: the clock on the wall, the prepackaged portion, the calories prescribed by a diet program, the foods we've been told are good for us . . . the bottom of a bucket of popcorn.

Multiple clinical studies suggest that mindful eating, a form of meditation in which you focus on the sensory cues of the eating experience without judgment, can be an effective way to increase our awareness of our innate biological hunger and satisfaction cues, helping reconnect us to our appetite and our body's need for different kinds and quantities of fuel.[1] If you've gotten into the habit of eating your meals on autopilot or letting your empty plate or package dictate when you're done, meditation practice can help you break free of those habits by allowing you to develop greater awareness of when you are truly hungry, and eating only then.[2]

Meditation helps you manage your energy level.

Another thing that meditation helps you recognize is your energy level, which is an excellent gauge of how well you're eating. Certain foods can set us up for first an energy spike and then an energy crash. (Learn more about specific food choices in chapter 6.) Having a regular meditation practice creates a mindful awareness of the experience in your body so that you notice how certain foods affect you, both when you're eating them and then several hours afterward.

After using this meditation practice for a while, you become able to shift your focus when you're eating. Instead of asking yourself, *What sounds good? What am I craving right now?* you start to ask, *How do I eat to heal myself? How do I eat to energize myself? What am I feeding the engine of my body, of my metabolism?*

By helping you key in to your experience in your body and your energy needs, meditation allows you to fine-tune your eating program to give you sustained energy throughout the day. For some people, that might be eating every three hours; for others, every five. But figuring that out is easier once you've gained observation skills and become better connected with all of your body's signals.

Meditation helps you experience more diverse flavors.

Another important benefit of meditation is that it helps you notice all the flavors, textures, smells, and visual delights in your food. People who are overweight are sometimes depicted in media as slaves to overactive appetites. However, as counterintuitive as it may seem, overweight people tend to have *under*reactive taste buds. Often those who are most tempted to overeat or eat lower-nutrition foods do so in part because they have trouble tasting flavors and therefore seek out more intense flavors to satisfy their sensory cravings. That sets up a downward spiral: We eat overly processed foods, which acclimate our taste buds to strong, artificially enhanced flavors, often to the point where we can no longer sense the subtle flavors of fresh vegetables, fruits, nuts, and other healthful foods.

That's why one of the hardest transitions for someone going from a diet of highly processed foods to one richer in whole foods is getting used to the more subtle tastes. Compared with heavily processed foods, vegetables can taste bland, and cravers talk about not enjoying such "boring" food. But meditation can retrain your palate to notice and appreciate the delicious subtleties of all foods—even in a bowl of kale! Once you become more attuned, you start to notice the crunch or the curly leaf of different varieties, or how one type is milder or more bitter than another. Or perhaps all apples once tasted the same to you—ho-hum. But with meditation, you start to notice and appreciate how each of the hundreds of varieties of apples has its own taste and texture.

Many of my patients have told me that meditation is what finally helped them understand the big deal about organically grown versus industrially grown foods. Now they can taste the difference—it's become as obvious to them as the difference between a vine-ripened tomato, warm from the summer sun, and a conventionally-grown/packed/shipped tomato that might have perfectly red skin but, underneath, has chalky white flesh and no flavor. When we meditate, these finer points of sensory experience start to reveal themselves to us, in greater and greater detail, making it much more enjoyable (and, therefore, easier) to transition to healthier food choices.

Meditation helps you pick healthy foods.

In addition to helping us internalize these sensory pleasures, meditation also helps keep our brain "on"—not zoned out—so we can remain aware of the long-term effects of the food we're about to put into our body. Sometimes we get carried away in the moment, when we're at a party or celebration, surrounded by temptations. Meditation helps bolster our brain's executive function, the high-level decision-making processes that help us make choices based on goals rather than cravings. This increased executive control that we gain from meditation is a big facet of our ability to better regulate what and how much we eat.[3] Remaining mindful around food makes it surprisingly easier to make those in-the-moment food choices that protect your future health rather than simply satisfy your unhealthy cravings.[4]

Meditation helps you stop yo-yo dieting.

One of the biggest pitfalls on the path to long-term weight loss and health are those frustrating ups and downs of yo-yo dieting—especially when your weight starts to head more up than down. We can get entranced by the latest trend and put all our energy into following the newest fast or hard-core fitness program. But while each of these may have healthy components, what your body and your metabolism need most are steadiness and reliability, to trust that you will be nourished. Your metabolism counts on that and anticipates it. All the ups and the downs of turning from one new diet to the next make it a lot harder for your body to settle into a healthier weight.

Imagine you're at your job and you just want to get your work done and go home, but you have a difficult boss. You never know what he's going to tell you to do; you don't know if you're going to show up to have him yell at you, ridicule you, or even fire you. Yet, on another day, he's sweet as pie and praising you to all of your colleagues.

That unpredictability would be really stressful.

Well, that's the same unpredictability your metabolism experiences with yo-yo dieting. Eventually, your body just exists in survival mode, constantly planning for attack. Rather than healing and repairing, taking care of the internal organs, and functioning well, your nervous system is on constant alert, awaiting a famine. That lack of consistency can have a profound effect on the adrenal glands, the thyroid, and reproductive hormone levels, which are probably the three biggest physiological factors in women's struggle to shed weight. (We'll discuss this more in the next chapter.)

I know it can be so tempting to go for big results, very quickly. But based on my experience of watching patients over longer periods, the most effective thing that you can do is incorporate small changes, things that you can do regularly to keep your body balanced and centered, into your lifestyle for the rest of your life.

Like a few minutes of meditation every day.

Meditation helps you spot the "oh, well" effect and strengthen your willpower.

A regular meditation practice can help us be mindful of many types of distorted thinking, such as this one: *Oh, well, I had one cookie, so I blew it for today—may as well finish the box.* If we allow this cognitive distortion—also known as the abstinence violation effect—to go unchallenged often enough, that "oh, well" reaction can become an entrenched, intractable reflex. This reinforced habit may then migrate into other areas of your life, stealing your discipline and making the achievement of any goal quite challenging.

Meditation can strengthen your willpower muscle by helping you short-circuit this cycle before it really gets going. When you start meditating, you start to learn how to recognize the triggering thought early (*I had one cookie*) and give yourself the space to examine your next inclination *(Is one cookie really that big a deal? If I have the rest of the box, how will I feel?)* before you give in. Eventually, with enough mindful practice, you can learn to catch that "oh, well" *before* you give in to the thought distortion, and have a chance to break the reactivity chain.

Meditation helps disrupt the self-criticism/ self-sabotage cycle.

As meditation helps develop your awareness of the running commentary going on in your mind 24/7, you may begin to notice how often you say mean stuff to yourself:

I'm craving sugar.
I'm weak.
I'm fat.
I failed.

Once you notice these unhelpful thoughts, you can begin to disengage from charged emotions, release these judgments, and simply seek information about these thoughts. You can sit with the thoughts to extract their hidden messages: *Oh, I'm craving sugar. I wonder why? Did I eat? Yeah, I ate my lunch. I feel like I've been eating balanced meals. What is it? Well, maybe it is because I'm having trouble with my spouse and craving companionship. Or maybe I'm stressed because of my kids acting out. Maybe it's work?*

The reason you're craving sugar could be anything— but the important part is simply noticing the craving. Then, the second stage is asking why.

Ultimately, you might decide to give in and have the candy bar. (And that's okay—your meditation practice will help you derive even greater joy from it, and will help prevent one candy bar from turning into a binge.) But the unraveling process is able to begin there *because* you noticed it. Mindfulness simply gives you the nonjudgmental space to ask yourself, *Is this really serving my best interest?*

Without consciously examining our habits, we can get stuck in a rut that takes focused effort to disrupt. Mindfulness allows us to notice the patterns that might block us from healthful habits, such as starting the day with a smoothie, eating meals regularly, or keeping up with our exercise program. We may start to see that negative thinking can be the worst habit of all, the linchpin habit that enables all other bad habits and requires conscious attention and consistent effort to address.

Meditation helps you stop using food to soothe your emotions.

Eating serves emotional needs for all of us—but some more than others. Up to 30 percent of the people enrolled in weight loss programs have struggled with extreme emotional eating. Mindfulness practice can help counteract emotional eating in several ways. Similar to the "oh, well" cognitive distortion I mentioned earlier, meditation can also make us more aware of emotional triggers and how they're connected to our eating patterns, helping us to interrupt the chain of reactions that can lead to emotional eating.

If you've struggled with emotional eating, you

might have experienced a cycle like this: You are triggered in some way—by looking at a fashion magazine, an unpleasant encounter at work, a fight with a loved one, or some other stressful situation. Once the negative emotion is triggered, you may feel powerless to stop it, and you may even feel a sense that it will keep escalating until you do something to reduce or resolve it. *This* is the moment when an emotional eater might reach for some chips or cookies to help herself calm down. What makes emotional eating so insidious is how effective it can be—it can *seem* to temporarily solve the problem by distracting you from your negative emotions, thereby relieving your immediate distress. The relief that you feel in that moment (not to mention the neurochemical effect of foods we gravitate toward in stressful moments— high-sugar, high-fat, high-carb foods) only serves to reinforce that cycle in your brain, so it becomes that much easier to fall into the next time.

If you repeat this often enough, what was once a less-than-advisable coping strategy soon becomes an entrenched habit that feels impossible to break. Yet, with daily practice, meditation can help you slow down these complex "overconditioned" emotional responses, creating a couple of points on the decision-making chain of reactivity where it can be interrupted—even right as you reach for the next mouthful of food.[5] Mindfulness is one of the best antidotes to emotional eating, helping you notice these emotions when they arise, so that you can watch the process and create the needed mental space for more helpful strategies.

Mindfulness helps you reduce binge eating.

The awareness you get from meditation can serve as a spotlight on your motivation to eat. You start to notice that maybe you're craving sugar because you're missing some sweetness in your life. Or you're missing some attention from your family members, or maybe it's because you didn't eat all day. Being aware of these emotional triggers helps you pause long enough to notice where the desire to eat comes from. Instead of just reaching right for the chocolate bar or salty pretzels, this practice teaches you how to interrupt that reactivity cycle.

But sometimes emotional eating can become entrenched and morph into binge eating—a more serious condition, but one that meditation has also been proven to help relieve. One pilot study at Indiana

State University found that seven sessions of group meditation helped cut binge episodes by almost two-thirds and significantly decreased participants' depression and anxiety.[6] Another study by the same group found that meditation helped obese binge eaters develop overall greater self-regulation and balance around eating, and sustained improvement in binge eating, even four months after the end of treatment. The more meditation the participants did, the researchers found, the better they fared on their recovery.[7]

People with binge eating disorder react intensely to social and emotional cues and often have long-standing habits. At the same time, they tend to be disconnected from their own internal cues, especially around feeling satisfied after eating. While some of this can be attributed to genetic differences, researchers believe more likely it is the disconnection from our own internal experience that creates these patterns of mindless eating.

With traditional diet programs, we may lose five or ten pounds really quickly—but their emphasis on a specific calorie restriction or "tricking" your body out of hunger further disconnects us from our internal signals. These external structures don't allow the personal flexibility or opportunity to relearn healthy habits, and they completely ignore the intensity of the cravings binge eaters experience.[8] Yet by helping us reconnect to those hunger and satisfaction signals, meditation can make all the difference in regulating eating habits as well as reducing depression and anxiety—which all can lead to healthy weight loss.[9]

Meditation helps you change long-held assumptions/beliefs about yourself.

No matter how much we want to change, one of the hardest things to budge is our own self-concept. The images we hold of ourselves are remarkably stable. This "cognitive conservatism" often means that we can behave in ways that support and sustain an image, no matter if it's good or bad or whether we do so intentionally. If you've been clinging to a poor self-concept for a while, you may be frustrated with your inability to break this bad habit—but please know that lack of change is just your inner self's bitter determination not to be destroyed.

We humans are an odd bunch; we'll cling to our self-image whether it's hurting us or not, and no matter what type of self-sabotage might be required to maintain it. The trick is to make this innate drive toward self-fulfilling prophecy work *for* you rather than against you.

Meditation can help you examine your own long-held beliefs about yourself, and question them: *Is this true? Am I really X, or is that just my perception of what my people thought when I was growing up? More important, do I want to stay like X?* If you start to loosen the vise grip of your negative self-concept and open yourself to the idea that you are a worthy person who deserves vibrant health and happiness, you can let those magical self-fulfilling prophecies do their work, guiding your behavior toward choices that support your new, healthier self-image. (A great number of the meditations, journal exercises, and daily intentions in the Meditate Your Weight plan were designed to tap in to this exact drive.)

Meditation helps shift your focus from self-deprivation to self-nurture.

The way we typically think about losing weight has always been "weight loss = torture." We somehow believe losing weight is something that must be "endured"; to be effective, it must be painful and unpleasant. Researchers believe this propensity for self-torture may be related to the stigma around extra weight: Overweight people are believed to be "wrong" in our culture, so they must be forced to do their penance.

Yet public health research has proven that shaming people into losing weight never works. Stigma is de-motivating and actually leads to greater relapse rates, depression, and severely compromised overall health. And it's not your imagination—that stigma has grown dramatically recently. One Yale study estimates that the stigma against people who are overweight increased by 66 percent between 1996 and 2006. Research has documented the stereotypes behind it, which include some extremely harsh words (*lazy, weak-willed, unsuccessful, unintelligent, lack self-discipline,* et cetera).

These words are hurtful and usually false. But that doesn't stop the person who might be carrying extra pounds from hanging on to those labels and internalizing them. And if you're not aware, that judgment can play like a soundtrack in your head, all day, every day.

But meditation is a perfect antidote. The more we become more aware of what's going on inside our heads, without judging it, the more we can start to notice those unhelpful automatic thoughts and emotional reactions, and the faster we can stop the cycle before it starts.

Believe this: You can't bully yourself into losing weight.[10] With *Meditate Your Weight,* we focus on learning how to accept and love ourselves, without the layers of judgment, anger, and feelings of unworthiness that society wants to heap upon us. We can give ourselves compassion and forgiveness. This self-compassion is the cornerstone of the book. To look, to accept, and to love—as is. We can shift into setting goals and work toward being healthy, but without this cornerstone, there's nothing secure to build on.

Repeat after me: *I recognize that, within this body, no matter where I am today, I am wonderful, lovable, amazing. I'm beautiful inside and out, and I deserve respect, love, and vibrant health, no matter what.*

Now let's take a look at how the miracle of meditation also changes the physical structure and functioning of your body and your brain while it's busy changing the messages of your mind.

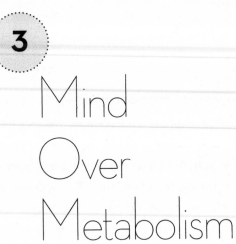

3

Mind
Over
Metabolism

Now that you've learned how the master habit of
meditation can help you overcome psychological
roadblocks, I'd like to talk about something that still
leaves me in awe, after so many years in this field:
how the practice can alter you *physically*.

Over the past several decades, dozens of research
centers around the world have studied the biological

effects of meditation, analyzing how it can change our physiology on a systemic, cellular, even genetic level. These changes have beneficial effects on many areas of our health, including the optimal functioning of metabolism and the regulation of body weight. In this chapter I'll talk about how meditation can help physically alter the shape, size, and functioning of your brain, rerouting the self-defeating neural patterns we talked about in chapter 2. (I geek out on the science a little, but bear with me—it's such cool stuff!) I'll also share how meditation has been proven to change your body's response to stress; to tone and soothe the autonomic nervous system; to reset an imbalanced endocrine system; to reduce systemic inflammation; and much more. And all of these physiological changes help to reboot your body's natural fat-burning settings, stabilize your metabolism, and allow you to achieve and sustain a healthy weight.

All this from a practice you can do in five to ten quiet minutes a day, with no expensive gear, starting today? That's pretty miraculous. Let's consider some of the many shifts meditation creates in the body, and how these changes help set you up for metabolic success.

Meditation changes your brain's reaction to stress.

Most of us think of stress as an unqualified negative. In normal conversation, "I'm stressed" would be considered synonymous with "I feel awful." But at its root, the experience of stress is neither good nor bad—the word *stress* simply refers to the mental and physical state we experience when we're faced with a challenge that pushes us beyond our normal limits. Our *reaction* to that challenge is what determines whether we experience this stress as a positive or negative thing.

A certain amount of challenge (or stress) can be very exciting. Looking forward to the birth of your first child. The rush of delivering a well-crafted presentation. Butterflies in your belly before a date with someone you really like. Each situation requires us to bring out our best, and a positive attitude toward these challenges helps us marshal all of our mental and physical resources—the increased energy, focus, and physical strength that come with the fight-or-flight response—to aid us in the task. Perhaps the single greatest benefit of meditation is its ability to shield us from the harmful effects of negative stress on the body and mind. In contrast to the fun "stress" of excitement and anticipation, chronic negative stress—worry and anxiety about a situation we feel is beyond our control—can increase muscle tension, irritability, headache, insomnia, high blood pressure, anxiety, depression, drug and alcohol abuse, overeating (or undereating), and many other unpleasant side effects. Left unchecked, prolonged negative stress can increase our risk for chronic inflammatory conditions of all kinds, including heart disease, obesity, stroke, diabetes, Alzheimer's, autoimmune conditions, and more.

The relentless hunger that leads to stress-induced overeating is just one of the issues that causes weight gain. Negative stress also elevates our blood sugar and causes us to become insulin resistant, or prediabetic. Our brains interpret stress as the body being in a state of famine, driving us to replace those lost calories as quickly as possible. That's why we tend to crave high-calorie, fatty/sweet/salty foods when we're stressed—our biochemistry is being manipulated by those stress hormone fluctuations and is crying out for more energy.

At the same time, stress mutes the reward system in the brain, driving us to consume larger and larger portions of these nutritionally bankrupt foods to trigger the dopamine response that will satisfy these stress-induced cravings. Every time we repeat this emotional eating cycle (discussed in chapter 2), the neurochemical balance and wiring in our brain further readjusts, nudging us toward ever-increasing quantities of food to find the same relief—the same pattern of increased tolerance seen in drug abuse.

Thankfully, meditation can help shield us from some of the dangers of negative stress. A study by researchers at the University of California San Francisco found that the more a group of stressed-out overweight women meditated, the greater their decreases in anxiety, markers of chronic stress, and belly fat—without any changes in their diet.[1] In another study, reported in the journal *Appetite,* researchers found that even among women with the largest cortisol response, those who underwent a brief meditation course reported less frequent reward-based stress eating and binge eating, and they lost more weight than women who'd not taken the class.[2]

Impressive, huh? But meditation's protective power isn't merely about relaxation or stress relief, and no amount of meditation can take away all the challenges in our lives. Instead, meditation works by changing our mental, emotional, and physiological *reactions* to those stresses. Research shows that simply changing our *beliefs* about stress itself can actually shield us from its harmful effects.

In the face of any stress, positive or negative, your body releases adrenaline and norepinephrine, both of which give you energy and focus your attention. Blood rushes out of your belly into your brain and your extremities, to gird you for the fight ahead, and you release more free fatty acids into your blood to fuel your efforts. If the challenge is met, you are flooded with the relief and sense of accomplishment that come from a hit of pleasurable neurochemicals, such as dopamine, your reward for a job well done. Then your adrenals release the hormone cortisol, the primary function of which is to return your body to homeostasis—taking blood and nourishment out of the brain and extremities and bringing it back to the belly, so you can "rest and digest."

When you look at a challenge and think, *I can do it! I've got this,* this positive reaction to stress is adaptive, building resilience and confidence. After you've celebrated and relished the success, your brain is armed with this positive memory, which will guide your attitude toward stress (and, thereby, your behavior) next time. Much as your muscles grow when you tax them in the gym, your capacity to meet and master challenges—your resilience—grows with every success. And this isn't just common sense—science has confirmed it. Researchers have found that individuals who have experienced a moderate amount of adversity show more resilience and a greater ability to meet challenges in the future.[3]

But what happens when you view stress as a negative? Well, the fight-or-flight hormonal cascade starts the exact same way, but there's a very critical moment when our attitude determines whether that stress will strengthen us and build our resilience capacity—or weaken us and break us down.

When you view stress positively, and you meet and master the challenge, your momentary burst of cortisol helps your system reset itself, and then it decreases—its job is considered done. But if you view that same challenge with the thought *I'm never going to be able to do that,* your adrenal glands will continue to release cortisol as long as you feel that fear. Your adrenals think you must not be done with the challenge yet, so they keep pumping out the cortisol, trying to bring you back to homeostasis.

This is why cortisol is sometimes termed "the hormone of defeat."[4] With repeated messages of *I can't do it,* and *I'm scared of what comes next,* your body releases a steady stream of cortisol that will increase the formation of fat cells—leading to toxic belly fat—as well as cause tremendous inflammation in the body, increase blood sugar (and the risk of diabetes), eat away at your brain and muscle tissue, suppress your immune system function, and much more.

Horrible, right?

But truly—and this is the part that still amazes me—all you need to do to avert this dangerous cascade is learn to stop yourself in that moment of doubt and fear. Rather than surrendering unquestioningly to the fear *(Stress is horrible, and I can't handle it!)*, you simply observe your stress *(Isn't this interesting? I am feeling stress.)*. If you can learn to just stop and consider your thoughts before you become engaged in them, you can head off the negative biochemical chain of events—and begin rewiring your entire nervous system.

A third of American adults believe that stress adversely impacts their health—but researchers are starting to get the word out that this *belief* is what is causing our stress problem, not the stress itself. In a landmark study, researchers at the University of Wisconsin reviewed the experiences and health-outcomes data of more than twenty-eight thousand people. After controlling for many factors, they found that those who'd reported both high levels of stress and a strong belief that this stress would cause health concerns had a 43 percent greater risk of premature death.[5] Compared with those who didn't believe that stress affected health, those who reported perceiving that stress affected health "a lot" were about four times more likely to be in poor health.

On the other hand, those who claimed to have tried stress-relief measures in the prior twelve months were less likely to report being in poor health. The act of attempting self-help indicates that these folks clearly believed that their level of stress was within their control, and that sense of personal agency helped them more than they may have consciously known.

It's clear: Our thoughts influence our lives. If we believe stress is bad for us, it will be; if we believe stress can be a good thing, it will be a catalyst to energize us and spur us into action. With a positive orientation, these feedback cycles build resilience, optimism, and confidence; with a negative one, the cycles damage our confidence, concentration, memory, immune system, emotional balance, relationships, careers—you name it, negative stress can make it worse. Every time we react to stress either with excitement or with fear, we trigger those positive or negative biological reactions—and prime our systems to repeat them next time.

Thankfully, we can put this innate feedback mechanism to work for us. We can learn to head off the negative stress response and reteach our brains how to react to stress, simply by committing to a daily session of meditation. This three-week plan is a gentle, easy way to get started and can open up a whole new world of mind-body benefits for you. And research proves it: You don't need more than a few minutes a day to start changing your brain.

A brain scan study on novice meditators conducted at Massachusetts General Hospital, the largest teaching hospital of Harvard Medical School, found that meditating for less than half an hour a day for eight weeks decreased the density of gray matter in the amygdala, an area of the brain known to play a role in fear, anxiety, and stress.[6] Previous studies found the reverse to be true as well: Trauma and chronic stress thickened gray matter in the amygdala, making it more sensitive and reactive to negative stimuli.

The degree of these changes was directly correlated to the participants' own reduction in perceived stress—the less stress they reported, the greater the reduction in the density of their amygdala. These brain scans also found increased gray-matter density in the hippocampus, a site of learning and memory that's often smaller in people with chronic negative stress, as well as increases in the size of the cerebellum, an area of the brain that helps us keep our emotions balanced. This study makes clear that regular meditation practice can directly *change* our brains and our personal experience of stress, not simply relieve it.

Once you begin meditating, you'll be more likely to approach potential stresses with a greater ease and with less internal conflict, greatly reducing the wear and tear on your body. By doing the three-week plan, research suggests you'll be well on your way to rewiring your entire nervous system to greet challenges with excitement, confidence, and resilience, clearing the path for a happier, more peaceful, and more rewarding life.

Meditation changes your nervous system's response.

If we're not yet tuned in to our internal conversations, we can remain oblivious to the reasons we feel so stressed all the time. And then add this: The moment

we walk out the door of any home in America—
blam!—we are blasted by a culture that thrives on
triggering the fight-or-flight response as often as possible.

Television, Internet, smartphones, 24/7 e-mails,
texting, social media—all these messages are com-
peting for our attention, looking for a foothold in our
psyche. For every media, the most effective way to
get us to pay attention is to wave a red flag in front of
our reactive amygdala and try to hijack the nervous
system. Think of meditation as a way of creating
Wonder Woman's force field around your brain—
you can see the stimulus, you can hear it, but it can't
touch your brain and your nervous system unless *you*
allow it to.

Our body's autonomic nervous system is actually
composed of two parts: the sympathetic and parasympathetic. The sympathetic nervous system is
the gas pedal, the hard-charging, deadline-oriented,
goal-directed side, the part that kicks into gear during the fight-or-flight response. As we discussed previously, we were never meant to stay in fight-or-flight
mode for more than a few minutes at a time—just
long enough to outsmart (or outrun) the immediate
danger.

Our bodies are actually meant to spend more time

in rest-and-digest mode, driven by our parasympathetic nervous system. The brake to the sympathetic system's gas pedal, the parasympathetic nervous system slows our heartbeat and breath, allowing blood to flow throughout the body once more, soothing the amygdala, and encouraging our bodies and brains to start doing all those essential-but-not-life-or-death actions: digesting food, repairing cells, making long-term plans, creating art, falling in love.

Think of our primitive selves (or of animals in the wild): Most of our days were relatively low-stress. We rose with the sun and slept under the moon. We stayed in gentle motion most of the day, foraging for the water and plants and nuts that could sustain us—calm, productive activity, with sporadic bursts of reward (a clump of extra-ripe raspberries!). We were generally not on the hunt (or being hunted) 24/7. This rest-and-digest mode allowed our bodies to be nourished, our organs to be healed, and our energy stores to be built back up for the next challenge. Of course, when we faced an emergency, the sympathetic mode was ready and waiting to pump the blood into our muscles to get us out of danger. But the majority of our time was always meant to be spent walking in the woods, looking up at the clouds, and being with our loved ones—that is, in parasympathetic mode.

Fast-forward to the twenty-first century, and if we're not conscious about the way we live our lives, our daily reality can become dominated by sympathetic activities. Take something we do every day, like driving. You drive a bit above the speed limit, because you're late getting the kids to school. You're hypervigilant about any sign of a police car—*don't want to get another ticket!* You get cut off, feel a quick burst of adrenaline—and then anger *(What a %&^$# jerk!)*. You catch a glimpse of your child sitting in the backseat, feel guilty for swearing. *(Am I a bad mother?)* Tell yourself that, yes, of course you are because you're taking your kid to daycare, which your mother-in-law has compared to child abuse. Take another swig of your twenty-ounce dark-roast coffee, which is all that got you out of bed this morning . . .

With a relentless foot on the accelerator of the sympathetic nervous system, we power through our days, gutting it out until the weekend, or our yearly vacation, thinking that this brief respite is going to make up for those hours upon days (upon years!) of adrenaline-fueled activity. But with repeated use, the sympathetic system switch can get stuck in the on position, and the parasympathetic system can weaken and atrophy. You can do all the right things with diet and exercise, but if your parasympathetic mode isn't functioning properly, your cortisol will remain high and your body will store more fat. We have to bolster our parasympathetic response so we can learn to relax our bodies as efficiently as we can stress ourselves out. Simply put: We need to build our relaxation muscles. Luckily, meditation is one of the best ways known to do just that.

This building of our relaxation muscles can happen on a moment-to-moment basis. Simply exhaling one long breath engages the parasympathetic system and can decrease our heart rate. If we can build in more of these moments throughout our day, one conscious moment after another, we can very quickly downshift our degree of reactivity. Meditation has been shown to increase the alpha waves in our brains (associated with focus and staying on task) as well as decrease our heart rate, respiratory rate, blood pressure, muscle tension, and activity in our amygdala.[7] Meditation practices downshift the activity of the hypothalamic-pituitary-adrenal (HPA) axis, reducing cortisol and other stress hormones, continually resetting our metabolism in response to various levels of stress. Meditation also increases beneficial hormones, such as DHEA and growth hormone, which help maintain lean body tissue, and thyroid stimulating hormone and prolactin, which help support a strong metabolism.[8] All of these changes continually reinforce one another, and by design, the Meditate Your Weight plan capitalizes on this combined effect.

By creating a framework that triggers these physiological changes, the program escorts your body into rest-and-digest mode, where it can begin to release excess weight. This ease, this relaxed approach to health, is something that our bodies can more easily and joyfully sustain over time, unlike taking deadly pills, doing extreme exercise, radically cutting calories, or any other extreme measures we may be tempted to try.

We really don't need to push. What we need to do is give our bodies a break.

Meditation tones your vagus nerve.

Consciously spending more time in parasympathetic mode strengthens the tone of our vagus nerve, which communicates messages between many critical body systems. When you hear people talk about getting a "gut reaction," they are partly referring to the actions of this tenth cranial nerve, which extends from brain stem to abdomen by way of multiple organs, including the heart, esophagus, and lungs. A core component of the parasympathetic system, the vagus nerve is triggered in times of stress, to help balance out our strong sympathetic nervous system reaction. Doctors can get a sense of our vagal function in the subtle increase of our heart rate when we breathe in (sympathetic function) and a subtle decrease when we breathe out (parasympathetic function). The difference between these two rates creates a ratio known as heart rate variability, an important indicator of cardiac health.[9]

Having good vagal tone suggests that you have flexible emotional responses to any strong stimuli— and it turns out to be one of the most reliable predictors of cardiac health, emotional resilience, and overall physical health. In contrast, low vagal tone has been linked to high inflammation, greater risk of heart attacks, and lower odds of survival after heart failure. Vagal tone is highest when we're kids; it's inherited from our parents and locked in with secure attachment to our primary caregivers. Without a lot of cardio exercise, vagal tone tends to drift down as we get older and really fall off with the development of heart disease or diabetes. Endurance exercisers— long-distance runners, swimmers, or cyclists—tend to have the best vagal tone as they age—but guess how else you can consciously strengthen the vagus nerve? You got it: by meditating.

In a study done at the University of North Carolina, researchers followed a group of sixty-five people for two months. After the trial they found that those who'd taken the compassion-focused "loving-kindness" meditation course had significantly increased their vagal tone. This type of meditation encourages you to feel compassion for yourself, your loved ones, your community, and even those with whom you are currently struggling. The researchers believe that using this meditation helped people focus on recalling positive emotions and experiences, which acted almost as "nutrients for the human body," strengthening the participants' relationships and boosting their vagal tone and parasympathetic health. The more time people meditated, the more pleasant their interactions with others became, reinforcing all the beneficial effects in what the researchers called "a self-sustaining upward spiral of growth."[10]

Meditation improves your metabolism-protecting sleep.

Another victim of our go-go-go culture is our nightly free fountain of youth, restorative sleep. You've likely been harangued by your doctor, your mother, and every publication on the planet to get a good night's sleep, so I don't need to remind you how important it is. Many of the beneficial physiological changes meditation creates in the body are similar to the changes that happen during sleep, with your body resting in parasympathetic activity during the slow-wave or "deep" phases of sleep. As we get older, we tend to spend more time in REM sleep, which is governed by sympathetic activity, and less in slow-wave. But research has found that meditation helps us retain our flexible nervous system response during different phases of sleep. Meditating also brings more blood flow to our frontal lobe during sleep, nourishing the site of our executive function for the next day's work. Melatonin, a hormone that helps us fall and stay asleep, increases with meditation as well—one unpublished study found that nighttime melatonin levels were almost five times higher in meditators than in non-meditating controls.[11]

In many ways, sleep and meditation both help tip

us into parasympathetic predominance. When we can fall asleep faster and get more restorative sleep, every single aspect of any weight management plan becomes easier and more pleasant.[12] Some who struggle with sleep issues may choose to do the daily meditations of this program at night (or add on a second session of meditation) to further ease the transition to sleep.

Meditation helps keep your body young.

We've talked about how meditation helps us relieve and even prevent negative stress, and the many physical and emotional benefits that flow from that. Now here's something amazing: Meditation appears to slow, or even reverse, the aging process.

You may have heard about telomeres, the protective caps at the ends of our chromosomes, the strips within cells that hold our DNA. The length of these telomeres is determined by many factors, especially age, and can degrade faster in cases of depression or chronic negative stress. When we obsess over stressful thoughts, we can keep our bodies in a perpetual state of reactivity that can shorten these telomeres, which has been associated with heart disease, diabetes, cancer, Alzheimer's disease, and osteoporosis. But mindfulness techniques can help manage those risks—and by shifting our perceptions from threats to challenges, decreasing anxious rumination, and dampening our systemic stress response, we are likely also protecting our telomeres.[13] That's important to our weight loss efforts because when telomeres work well, they support the activity of the mitochondria—our cells' powerhouses, which help us turn food into fuel—as well as allow our bodies to burn stored fat as fuel.[14]

One study of seventy breast cancer patients showed how powerful an impact meditation can have on telomere length. The women were divided into three groups—meditation class, group therapy, and a control group—for eight weeks. Researchers found that those who'd participated in the mindfulness class or the group therapy both had protected the length of their telomeres during the eight weeks; the control group's telomeres had shortened.[15] An analysis of a group of well-respected scientific studies on 190 participants revealed that meditation had increased telomerase, the enzyme that influences telomeres' length, in immune system cells.[16]

Other research suggests that the length of time

necessary for meditation to change your genetic expression might be as short as *one day.* A study sponsored by the National Center for Complementary and Integrative Health tested the genes of meditators and non-meditators and found that those who'd meditated for an average of three years could change the expression of several genes related to inflammation and stress recovery in a single day, after a prolonged meditation session.[17]

The science continues to develop in this area, but this kind of research just blows me away. Sitting on your cushion for a brief time every day can help you protect your health and well-being on a *genetic* level. That's powerful.

Meditation improves your brain—and then your entire life.

When your body is balanced, when your internal organs are functioning well and all parts of your body do what they're supposed to do—that's when your metabolism will hum along happily and weight loss should become much easier. But first we have to disabuse ourselves of a deprivation mentality when it comes to our weight. We seem to have this idea that metabolism is this separate entity that we have to *train*—we have to put it through the paces, tightly control what we're eating and how we're exercising. But in reality, your health *is* your metabolism—it's all connected. If you get the body and the organs functioning optimally, really make health your focal point, the metabolism part will come, not to worry.

The best part of approaching your health from a place of bounty and ease—as opposed to deprivation—is that these changes tend to be the ones that stick. When you deprive yourself and do intensive diets, then regain the lost weight, the impact of this yo-yo effect is actually much worse on the metabolism long-term than simply remaining at a constant weight. Bottom line: This approach is not working. A large body of research tells us that overweight folks who lose weight tend to regain about half of it back within the first year. Eight out of ten obese people who lose weight return to their original weight—or exceed it—within three to five years.[18]

We need a different approach. We need to go more slowly, get away from the traditional approach to dieting, and retrain ourselves to look at a different long-term picture.

Changing the focus to this long-term perspective has wonderful side benefits as well. You start to feel better, and those little symptoms you wouldn't necessarily go to the doctor for—the poor sleep, the lagging energy, the constant low-grade headaches, even the emotional balance—all start to smooth out and resolve on their own. As the body functions better, everything starts feeling better. Especially your mind.

Where to begin? Simply by being kinder to yourself.

We talked about self-compassion in chapter 2. Turns out self-compassion doesn't just help you stick to your intentions—it helps improve your physical and emotional health, too. A joint University of North Carolina/University of Michigan study found that seven weeks of compassion-based meditation training increased the participants' daily experiences of joy, gratitude, and hope. As the participants did more meditation, the effect strengthened. They also felt more connected with and supported by their friends and loved ones; they had greater self-acceptance; they felt more certain about their unique purpose in life, and they were more satisfied with their lives. Again—all that for a few short minutes a day?

Researcher Paul Gilbert, famous for his work in

compassion therapy, likens the practice of training the mind to tending a garden.[19] Left to its own devices, your brain *will* change, just like a garden will grow without human intervention—but who knows what'll end up in there? Certainly not well-tended tomatoes or gorgeous roses. Most likely, your garden will be overtaken by weeds and brambles, which may choke out the plants you prefer. But if you take the time to tend your garden, even just five minutes a day, you will see a major difference in which plants live and die, what flowers falter and what flowers thrive.

Meditation is tending your own interior garden, and a small amount of focused effort will yield beautiful results, much more pleasing than simply taking your chances with what sneaks in and takes over.

SIT DOWN, YOU'RE READY

You've learned all about the psychological and the physiological effects of meditation and how it can help you lighten up inside and out. Now it's time to learn the basics—the what, where, and how of meditation—so you can jump in and start experiencing these benefits for yourself.

YOUR 21-DAY RETREAT

Part 2

4

Establishing Your Daily Practice

Now that you have a better understanding of why meditation is so powerful, you can start to use it to help resolve some of your long-standing challenges.

During the 21-day retreat, we'll spend time each day thinking about some of the biggest hurdles to optimal weight. We'll consider:

How do these issues really apply to your life?

How can you use meditation to take a deeper look at them, and consider all of their implications?

How have they shaped your physical and emotional health to this point?

How will you use them to grow from here?

By the end of the 21 days, you'll have a deeper understanding of some of the issues that may have held you back in the past. You'll also have more compassion for yourself, and the greater ease, confidence, and effectiveness that brings, as well as a map for a gentle, sustainable, peaceful path forward.

First, let's talk about the specifics of the daily practice. Once you finish gathering a few materials together and reading through the basics, you'll be ready to start.

HOW OFTEN TO MEDITATE

Developing a regular routine is the most important thing to do when you begin meditating. Frequency is far more important than duration, as it helps your nervous system create a consistent pattern. Based on my patients' experiences, the more frequently you can follow that pattern, the more helpful (and long-lasting) the benefits will be. As we go through the program, the duration of your meditations will change, but the routine is really what's most important. At least for these 21 days, please aim for daily practice—even if you can only meditate for three minutes.

Everyone's ideal time of day will be a little bit different. Pick a time that works for you. I love the morning, and I think I'm not alone—there's something magical about taking advantage of the early morning, first thing. Take a few minutes to wake up, maybe walk around a bit. I try to meditate within thirty minutes of waking up—before my mind starts thinking, before the computer is on, before I start reviewing what's on my to-do list.

Some have trouble meditating before coffee. If you find you keep falling back asleep, go ahead and have a cup before you begin. (You may soon find you don't need it!) If morning doesn't work for you at all, you could try right after work. Or even right before bed. There's no right or wrong time, no specific moment that's more effective than another—as far as the nervous system goes, the timing is irrelevant.

What's most important is finding a realistic, regular time you can commit to. (Note: In the day-by-day instructions, I assume you're meditating and doing your journal exercises in the morning and that you'll carry your intentions throughout the day. If you meditate at a different time, you can adjust these instructions to fit your own rhythms and preferences.)

HOW LONG TO MEDITATE

If you already have a meditation practice, you can either substitute this program or add it to your existing practice. If you're just starting out, don't be afraid to *think small*. Seriously. Consistency is the key here, so remember that a short meditation every day is far superior to a longer meditation once a week.

Here's a sample meditation schedule for someone who is just starting (or getting back into) daily practice:

Days 1 to 3: 3 minutes

Days 4 to 9: 5 minutes

Days 10 to 15: 7 minutes

Days 16 to 20: 10 minutes

Days 21 forward: 12 minutes

This is just a guideline, a good starting point to create a habit and train the brain. Increase the amount of time spent meditating when you feel you're ready. The best way to increase is when you *want* to do so (versus feeling like you *have* to).

Note that these times are for the meditation portion of the program; afterward we will spend time each day writing in our journal.

WHERE TO MEDITATE

We sometimes get the message that meditation has to be done in this perfect, serene environment. Now, don't get me wrong—of course it would be great if we could all have a room where we can shut the door and bliss out in peaceful silence. But most of us don't, so we create the best situation we can with the tools we have.

If possible, find a small space where you can set up a mini sanctuary for yourself—perhaps it's on the floor in front of a low table with some pictures of loved ones, or a candle, or just a memento of something that makes you happy. When you dedicate a space to meditation, each time you go there your brain will get the signal that it's time to de-stress. Try to find a place away from your computer, to-do list, phone, and anything else that gets your mind revving.

If you can't create a permanent space, just find a place that allows you to feel remote for that time, as far as possible from distractions. Some people actually like to meditate in the workplace because it helps them bring a relaxed vibe into the work space. For others, the hum of the workplace makes their mind wander even more, so that doesn't work for them. Some people love meditating in their bedroom because it feels more relaxed; others, it puts to sleep. There can be a very fine line between emptying the mind and falling asleep or between being consciously alert and too distracted by the computer sitting next to you and all the things that you know you have to do.

Once you've established your personal place for your meditation routine, you may find that you want to meditate in other areas as well, but at least for a few weeks you will find it much easier to slip into the mind-set of meditation if you go to the same place every day. You can also keep all your needed materials in one place, creating less opportunity to become distracted or otherwise pulled away from your practice. You may need to do a little bit of experimentation, but once you have a spot, claim it wholeheartedly: *my meditation spot.*

A Note to Parents of Small Children

Most parents I know would love to be in a place where they can shut the door and know their kids will not disturb them during meditation time. But let's be honest here: That's probably not going to happen.

As a parent, you've probably come to grips with knowing that a certain level of chaos is inescapable. Try to stay away from the misconception that you have to find the perfect space or the perfect time. At some point, you're probably going to get disturbed, and it's not the end of the world. Just start, and even if you get distracted, even if you have to stop in the middle, even if your kids barge in on you and there's some emergency that you have to attend to—well, at least you've done part of your meditation. Finding your peace amid the din will simply be another element of your practice.

GETTING INTO POSITION

You have a few options when selecting how to sit. It's a matter of personal preference. Probably the hardest thing about meditating is sitting. Our backs get sore. Our hips are tight. It's very difficult to get comfortable. If you have flexible hips, or maybe you have a yoga practice, it might be more comfortable for you to sit on the floor.

Sitting on the floor: Sit with your legs crossed and tuck a cushion under your bottom. (See "Pick Your Sitting Tools," page 98.) You want to have the hips up just slightly higher than the knees, mainly so you can sit upright more easily for the comfort of your spine. If the knees are higher than the hips, your low back tends to round and your upper back starts to feel really tight. (When this happens to me, I'll feel it in my whole back, which screams at me while I'm trying to sit quietly.) A certain amount of discomfort is inevitable, but stacking the spine will decrease that as much as possible.

Sitting in a chair: Sitting in a chair can minimize the pressure in your back and hips so you can have a more pleasant experience. However, it's easy to slump down and get *too* comfortable, so help yourself stay alert. Sit on the end of the chair so that your feet are on the ground and your spine is still upright.

If there's a medical or personal reason why that won't work for you, you can sit against the back of the chair, but you want to make sure that you're not leaning back so much that you're dozing off (or even just zoning out).

Lying on your back: If neither of those positions works, you can lie on your back. The hard thing about lying on your back is the very natural tendency to fall asleep or zone out. You do want to get clear in the mind, true—but you're aiming for *conscious* alertness.

Clearly, there are pros and cons to each position: Sitting upright allows you to stay more alert and makes the mental part of it easier. Lying down is easier on the back but much harder for staying conscious and alert. Sitting on a chair can be that "just right" middle ground, especially for new meditators.

Pick Your Sitting Tools

You will need only a few simple tools. Some of these help you to complete the exercises; most help you relax during your meditation and take the pressure off of your hips or knees. You needn't get all of these—experiment until you find those that work for you.

Meditation stool: Some meditation stools allow you to sit with your feet tucked underneath, so that you can meditate in a kneeling position without putting too much weight on your heels. Other types of stools support your back while you are sitting cross-legged or in lotus position.

Yoga block: If you don't have a meditation stool, you can sit in the same position using a standard-size yoga block placed between your legs and under your bottom, so you can kneel without hurting your knees. (You can cover it with a blanket or towel, for softness.)

Meditation cushion: Sitting cross-legged

on a round or long cushion specifically designed for meditation can help you get your
hips at the right height—just slightly higher
than your knees. (Note: Meditation pillows are quite dense, to support your body
weight without collapsing; regular pillows
are typically not firm enough.)

Rolled-up blanket or towel: If you can't or
don't want to purchase a meditation cushion, the next best thing can be a firm blanket or a towel, as they are usually thick and
dense, so they're perfect for this purpose.
(And they're always easy to find, even when
you're on the road in a hotel.) Simply fold
or roll the blanket or towel to the desired
height for your back and hips.

Timer: I recommend setting a timer before you begin to meditate—doing so will
free you from concerns about losing track
of time. The timer on my phone works well
for me. Putting your phone on airplane
mode or do-not-disturb mode will ensure
that you don't receive any calls or texts

while you meditate. Consider downloading a mindfulness bell app for a soothing signal at the end of your meditation. With a timer, you don't have to worry about going over, or not staying in meditation long enough, or opening your eyes and trying to figure out how long it's been. Just set the timer and you're off.

Journal: Find a journal that pleases you—lined or unlined, hard- or softcover, large or small. What's most important is that you like how it looks and feels, and it inspires you to be honest with yourself and your feelings.

When you're sitting, whether on the floor or in a chair, you want your posture to be upright, the spine erect, resting your hands in two different ways.

1. *One hand on top of the other, with palms facing up.* One of the primary posture goals is to get the shoulders and the upper back to be as comfortable as possible. Whether placing one hand upon

the other feels comfortable will depend on your arm length, your torso length, and where you want to rest your arms. Resting one hand on top of the other can relieve tension in the shoulders for some, but you'll need to experiment and find what's comfortable for you.

2. *Resting hands on your thighs.* The best way to gauge where to place your palms in this approach is to notice where your elbows hang. Ideally, they'll be right underneath your shoulders. If you have your hands all the way out on your knees, it may be more difficult for your shoulders to relax. Bending your elbows allows them to drop under your shoulders, so your shoulders can relax, which allows your chest to open and your neck to relax. In this position you can turn the palms up or down, depending on what feels more helpful. Traditionally, palms down is a more grounding technique, helpful if you feel anxious or have a restless mind, and palms up can be a more receiving position, for times when you

feel more drained or fatigued. You can pick one and stick to it or change it as needed.

Now, is any of this 100 percent restful? No. The reality is that your muscles still have to be engaged to hold you up, so you'll never be completely relaxed

A Word About Discomfort

Some discomfort is natural. A part of the work of meditation is the process of being able to observe some of that discomfort and be okay with it. Noticing discomfort in meditation is a reflection of the discomfort our minds contend with in the rest of our lives. But if you are experiencing a significant amount of pain or any sharp, intense pain, it may be a good nudge to check in with your doctor (or other physical medicine expert, such as a physiotherapist, acupuncturist, yoga therapist, physiatrist, or someone similar) to see if there is something that needs to be addressed.

while you're sitting. But by consciously arranging your body, you're able to position yourself with the least resistance to gravity and the least tension in your neck, back, and shoulders. If there's another position that works for you, that's fine, too. As long as your position is comfortable, helps you relax, and allows you to stay alert, you'll be ready to meditate.

HOW TO MEDITATE

I'll instruct you on meditation throughout the book, but let's start here with a few basics about meditating for the Meditate Your Weight retreat.

Before you begin each day, read through the day's introduction and the description of the meditation. Then close the book and put it aside. Settle yourself in your meditation spot. Relax your body as much as possible. Set your timer (if you use your phone, make sure it's on airplane mode) and put it nearby.

Then close your eyes. Recall the instructions from that day's meditation, and begin.

Once you begin to meditate, you may notice your breath at first. We might notice that our breathing is a little choppier than we want it. Maybe we have this idea that our breath should be smooth and even and deep. Our mind suddenly starts thinking and making judgments.

That process of mentally drifting off happens almost immediately, even after one breath. The essence of meditation is simply being able to watch that drifting, that wandering, that wondering—but not become engaged in the thoughts themselves. Whether you've been meditating for years or decades or days, that wandering is going to happen. But being able to notice it, and remind yourself to bring your focus back into the present moment, *is* meditation. You are strengthening the muscles of the mind.

When we notice our minds being caught up with thoughts and distractions, we begin to notice the connection between the mind and how our thoughts make us feel. Often, these thoughts and their connections will change our breath and our heart rate. Again, come back to that process of just noticing how these thoughts affect us—noticing the changes in our body as we respond to our thoughts. This process helps you learn to "flip the switch," catching yourself before you fall into a sympathetic nervous system response and tipping yourself back into your parasympathetic mode.

For example, when I first sit down in meditation, my inner narrative might go something like this: *Okay, I'm sitting. Now I'm breathing. Now my breath is choppy, and I wish it was a little less choppy. I wish my breath was smoother. I wish my breath was deeper. I know how important the breath is. I know how important this is to my health. And I have to breathe deeper because I remember seeing that study yesterday on the Internet and how important it is for me to sit here.*

At that point I might realize suddenly that my mind has wandered off. (And I've been doing this for many years!)

I try to handle it all gently. Instead of judging myself for having a thought, I mentally "laugh"—*oh, you silly brain, there you go again*—and then I bring my mind back to my breath and the topic of my meditation.

This practice of becoming an observer, learning to watch and not get involved, transcends meditation. To be able to see our lives, our friends' lives, our family members' lives, and not get involved—takes practice. We need conscious awareness to gently resist our tendency to want to get involved, to start to shift things, to give advice. It's not that we shouldn't want to help others with their challenges—of course we do. But the difference is how we do that. When we become observers, we're less reactive; we're able to step back, watch, and take things in first, then move forward into intentional action. Instead of leaping to conclusions or knee-jerk reactions, we can enlist the frontal lobe, consider all the evidence, and make good choices. You gain such clarity when you become an observer—and you also become a really good listener, which is most of what your friends and loved ones want anyway (more than unsolicited advice).

AFTER YOUR MEDITATION

When the timer goes off or the bell rings, take a minute to finish, just watching your breath. When you're ready to open your eyes, go ahead. Then grab a pencil and start your Mind Makeover journaling exercises.

It's very important that you do not read the journal prompts before you do the day's meditation. Just read to the end of the meditation, stop, and immediately set the book aside while you do the meditation. That may be difficult—your instinct may be to keep reading. But you want your mind to be focused on the here and now, not already thinking about what you're going to write in your journal.

Once you're done with the journal exercise, you'll review your daily mantra (a mantra is not inherently spiritual—it is merely a word or a sound that you can repeat to help you concentrate) and your intentional awareness practice (a virtual lens through which you can choose to view the day's events). You might want to write down both on three-by-five-inch note cards to carry with you, so you can periodically remind yourself of the theme for the day.

Come back to those reminders as often as possible throughout the next twenty-four hours, even if it's just for a few moments, and enjoy the rest of your day. The next morning, or at your designated meditation time, come back to your meditation spot and repeat the process for the next day. Repeat for a total of 21 days, and you'll see many of the core reasons we struggle with our weight and our health; you'll gain insights into what has held you back in the past; and you'll have some truly useful ideas for how to move yourself forward. At the end of the three-week cycle, you will have established a very solid meditation practice, one that can carry you into your future.

So, are you ready? Gather your materials, select your spot, designate your time, and let's get started.

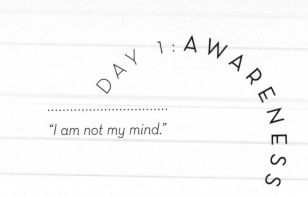

DAY 1: AWARENESS

....
"I am not my mind."

Today is the first day of your first cycle of the Meditate Your Weight program.

In the same way you can train your body's muscles at the gym, you can build your mind's strength and awareness on the meditation cushion. Day 1 is all about creating the foundation of good meditative practice, just like you would when you go to the gym to learn good form.

In chapter 1 I compared the temptation to engage in our own thoughts to parents who can't stop themselves from getting involved with their kids' lives as they watch them run up against any of the dozens of challenges they may face in the day (*Can I get that for you? Do you need help? Let me zip you up.*). And I'm sure you've felt that impulse even if you don't have kids. When a friend or a loved one encounters an issue or a problem, our automatic instinct is to jump in and help, show them how it *should* go (or even just *could* go).

When you begin to meditate, you'll quickly observe this tendency in yourself. You'll be amazed how often you feel your brain yearning to solve problems or concerns as soon as they float into your consciousness. But just as we need to learn to trust our kids (or our friends) to figure things out for themselves, we have to trust that those thoughts can take a breather while we're in meditation.

Learning to be an observer may sound like a simple process, but it's definitely not easy. The whole purpose is to teach ourselves to witness how our brains react to things we do notice, so we can start to understand how much of our lives is really unconscious. Thousands of details fly by us every day that we don't notice—which, on the whole, is a good thing, because our nervous systems would be overwhelmed otherwise. We wouldn't be able to process anything or get anything done if we had to filter every single thing. But many of those thought patterns that we keep on autopilot can affect us without our knowledge. In one sense, we are little robots marching through our lives based on unconscious computer code installed during our childhood. But on the other side, our conscious brains overcorrect so that we're in a constant churn of cerebral rumination about our past, our future—anywhere but here. What we're missing in this is a nice, centered, visceral, full-sensory experience of the now.

In the Buddhist tradition the distracted brain is referred to as the monkey mind, which always gives me a mental picture of a monkey in a cage, hopping around, rattling and shaking the cage. That monkey is just plain nuts. And, truthfully, if we were to write down every single thought that went through our heads as we sit, it *would* sound ridiculous. As we learn to step back and observe those thoughts, we can start to tell ourselves, *Huh, this really is wacky. My mind can take me off on crazy rants and raves just like a monkey in a cage going nuts, or a dog chasing its tail. That's just my human nature. This is what happens. I don't need to suppress it. I don't need to change it. But I want to be able to look at it and watch it so that I can start to be an observer.*

The more you practice, the more able you will be to laugh at these tangents, loosening your attachment to those thoughts and your compulsion to suppress them or control them. Just being aware of them will allow you to be lighter in your practice, rather than really serious and rigid and forcing. When we can learn to laugh at the reality of our monkey mind, we weaken the bondage of our minds controlling us, softening the grip of that constraint that we put on ourselves as adults having to be responsible all the time.

We don't have to be grown-ups right now. This is our time. And 3 minutes is all it takes to get started.

The challenge in today's practice is twofold. First we want to work on your ability to just watch your breath and not get involved. For most of us, it goes against our natural tendency. We try to make the breath more smooth or regulate the pace or depth. But in this practice you want to try to watch your natural breathing without changing it.

The second part of the challenge is attempting to stay present. In this meditation you may find yourself losing your place twenty or thirty times before you remember to come back. This is perfectly normal and part of the process. Your job is to keep coming back as you notice the natural tendencies of your mind to wander off on tangents. This simple technique trains the mind to focus on the moment-to-moment process of the breath and teaches us to be present. When you notice you have wandered off, try not to judge yourself; know this is natural, and just bring your awareness back.

Begin by finding a comfortable posture, and place your palms comfortably in your lap or on your knees. If you are sitting, make sure your hips are elevated slightly above the knees, with your elbows hanging under your shoulders.

Close your eyes or keep your eyes slightly open and softly focused toward the floor in front of you. (Experiment with both and see what feels best for you.) Then tune in to the inner landscape of the body. Just as you would notice the world around you with its sights and sounds and stimuli, bring that focus within you. Notice the quality of your breath and the movements that it creates, without trying to change it or control it. Notice all of the qualities—the sounds, the textures, the movement, and the natural pace—of your breath.

You may want to change the breath or make it longer. You may judge it: *Oh, it should be more evenly paced or it should be smoother.* But try instead to simply watch and notice it without trying to change it.

If you're new to meditating, these 3 minutes might feel like the longest 3 minutes of your life. Again, remember: You are doing it right. Just notice if it's hard or easy rather than worrying about how long it is. Notice as those thoughts come up, *Is it hard? Is it easy? Does it feel long? Does it feel short?* Notice any thoughts or sensations.

When your timer goes off, slowly shift your focus back to the room and open your eyes. You did it; you meditated. Pretty simple, right?

Now begin your Mind Makeover exercises.

Mind Makeover

When you are done meditating, settle into a comfortable sitting position to do your journaling. Most people find it helpful to come out of meditation and immediately reach for their journal as opposed to getting up and moving to another location to do the writing. Do not censor yourself or second-guess your responses; they are for your eyes only. Simply observe and record your responses to the following points.

1. What came to mind while you meditated? Any thoughts? Any sensations? Did it feel

long? Short? Were there emotions that came up? Did you feel fidgety? Jot down anything that you felt, and all of your thoughts.

2. Did you notice yourself judging the experience of your first meditation, your ability to pay attention, your ability to sit, to observe? Write down all of those judgments, unfiltered.

As soon as you're finished writing, close your journal and read "Today's Mantra" and the "Building Awareness" for day 1. Typically, a mantra is a statement—and for most days of the Meditate Your Weight program, they will be. But today I ask a question to help you open up and develop a receptive mind state. Copy the mantra out on a note card to carry with you, or simply write it in your journal to help remember. Try to come back to this mantra at least two or three times, or as often as you think of it, throughout your day today.

....

TODAY'S MANTRA:

What does the experience of living in my body feel like right now?

....

Building Awareness

The mind-body connection can be really beneficial, but it can also be really limiting. We work so much on reconnecting the mind and the body in a way that's healthy and useful, but when the mind and the body get too intertwined, it's difficult to separate them. You are not your mind; you are not your body. You are both, and more. We need to strike the right balance in connecting the mind and the body in a way that allows you to still be cognizant of the two as separate entities. Appreciating this difference can help you realize that you're not a slave to any reactionary response, whether emotional, mental, or physical. You have the ability to broaden that gap between the initial stimulus and your reaction to it.

Also, while many people talk about letting go of judgments, remember that the key is to just notice them. (As a perfect example of why this is important, remind yourself of the research you read about in chapter 3: Stress itself is not at all unhealthy—rather, it is our beliefs, our *judgments,* about stress being unhealthy that make it dangerous for us.)

Today, notice when you have a stressful situation. (Most of us have at least one—often many more—per day.) Notice how your body responds and what sensations it creates. Notice how that stress response affects you. One of the nice things about meditating is getting in touch with that inner landscape of the body. Notice how just dropping into that awareness changes what you feel.

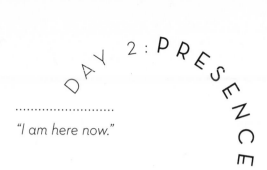

DAY 2: PRESENCE

"I am here now."

Today we are building on the practice you began on day 1. We're learning how to watch the mind's process and laugh at its monkeying around. We're noticing our human tendencies and developing awareness around just watching the breath. We're getting more intimate and familiar with the inner workings of the mind.

As we talked about yesterday, it is human nature for the mind to wander. Our ability to laugh at that and be okay with that aspect of our nature is a really important part of training the nervous system.

In my experience, one of the key factors in weight loss is our ability to notice the whole experience—to be able to find a state of health by watching how our body responds to different foods or movements, and how this state of health helps the metabolism find its own balance. Losing weight doesn't necessarily have to be a heavy thing, like *I'm going to eat* this many *calories* or *I'm going to do* this much *exercise*. Instead it can be as simple as *I'm going to focus on noticing the experience in my body when I eat and when I move.*

Tuning in, without judgment, allows us to simply gather information about the body's experience:

> Am I feeling lethargic because I've been sitting all day?
> Do I need to get out and exercise?
> Am I feeling sleepy because I ate too much?
> Do I need to drink water? Do I need a lighter dinner?

These early days of meditation are planting the seeds of this practice of noticing what's going on in your body. We do this to create a sense of focus and to reestablish health as our focal point, knowing that a more smoothly running metabolism will come from that.

That's why day 2 is about presence. There's a difference between true presence and zoning out. We all know what it feels like to zone out—you're tired at the end of the workday, and you literally just sit back in your chair and daydream. Your head is empty.

During meditation, you're not zoning out—you are letting your mind be present and observe what happens in the stillness. You maintain awareness of your body and of whatever is happening, without judgment—being able to laugh at it, being able to watch it as it passes by. The mind will still wander, meander, roam—developing *presence* allows you to constantly come back.

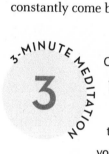

3-MINUTE MEDITATION

3

Get into your meditating position, set your timer, and begin.

Today your meditation is about tuning in to your inner landscape. As you sit, notice body sensations, bring your awareness to those sensations, and to your thoughts and feelings, without trying to change them.

Start with the breath itself, specifically at the nose. Notice all of the sensations that the breath creates in and around the nose. Notice the streaming of the breath inside of the nose. Notice the temperature of the outside of the nose. Notice where the breath enters and leaves the nose. Notice how the breath travels between the lip and the nose and over the upper lip. Keep your eyes soft under your closed eyelids. Remember that this is not a visual tracking, it's more an experiential, inner gaze.

Today's meditation is really just about getting comfortable being able to sit and notice the sensations of the breath, and just staying there for 3 minutes.

Mind Makeover

Today, for your journaling exercise, notice your experience:

1. How is your body feeling right now? Is your energy low?

2. How does the overall feeling in your body affect your experience right now? If you have low energy, or if you had poor sleep, or if you're feeling angry or stressed—how does that affect your experience?

3. How would your day be different if you were able to be more present with your family, your work, or yourself even for just 5 or 10 minutes?

....

TODAY'S MANTRA:

I am here now.

....

Building Awareness

Today you are drawing awareness to your presence. If you go to work, notice how your ability to be present in what you do affects your efficiency. If you live with your family, notice when you greet them how being fully present with them can affect the depth of your connection. As you tuck yourself in for sleep tonight, notice how your connection to yourself through the day can affect how you feel as the day comes to an end.

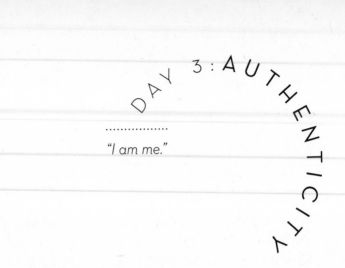

DAY 3: AUTHENTICITY

....

"I am me."

Authenticity is a big buzzword these days. But what does it really mean? At its root, being authentic is about being who you really are. But how do we define that? Is it in relation to someone else? Or through someone else's eyes?

Today, rather than default to seeing yourself the way you *think* others see you—a thought about a thought!—I want you to notice how you truly see yourself in the world, within your family, work, and relationships. You're going to look at your current self-image without judging it or trying to change it or wishing it away—you're just going to observe.

Why is this important? One of the most limiting factors in people's ability to get to that optimal health or weight—especially when they've already been doing "all the right things"—is their inability to change how they see themselves. I think this is often the most important, biggest block.

Our reality is created and re-created from moment to moment, based on our perceptions of ourselves and the world around us. How do we see ourselves? We may have images of ourselves as fat or smart or serious, as funny or flaky or uptight—all different ways of viewing ourselves that aren't necessarily positive or negative. Once we look at how we see ourselves, we can come to recognize how these images can potentially block the body's ability to process the goals and visions that we have for ourselves.

Seeing yourself as you are doesn't need to have anything to do with your dreams for the future. And much as we believe it does, our current state doesn't necessarily have anything to do with our past or the events that brought us to the present.

For today, I just want you to notice that reality is created and re-created every moment. Our reality is really just our perception. Acknowledging this elemental fact will help us internalize the truth: If you can change your mind-set, you can change your reality—and obviously you can change your life.

For many of us, the tendency is to see only the negative about ourselves or our situations. Maybe a slow metabolism, or a suspicion of a not-so-high IQ. Maybe a pattern of not following through on projects, or of not being there to help a friend in need. But at the same time, we also have our strengths: Good taste in movies and music. Love of family. Being able to laugh at ourselves. Recognizing our strengths, even as we try to address our weak points, can be difficult.

This is where meditation can help: Seeing yourself from an observer's perspective helps you take in the whole picture. You develop the ability to detach and just say, *Okay, what am I?*

> I am smart.
> I can be a bit clumsy.
> I can read really quickly.
> I'm not very strong.
> I'm really funny, when I want to be.
> I'm curvy.

Everyone has a mixture of strengths and weaknesses. Today I'll ask you to use your observer mindset, take a good look at yourself, and say, *Okay, what am I?* But without the judgment.

I realize this may be a bit difficult—you've only been meditating for 2 days. That's totally understandable. As you try this, notice if it is harder for you to look at the negative or the positive aspects of yourself, and see if you can round out the view, even a little bit more.

Above all, as you go through this day's work, be gentle with yourself.

Begin by just noticing how you sit and how you hold yourself. Maybe specifically look at the positioning of your shoulders and your head. As you sit, you might notice your shoulders rolling forward and the closing off of your chest. Notice if your head dips forward or your chin juts out. Even notice how that affects your comfort in your low back and hips, or in your seat, your pelvis, or your legs. Noticing how you sit is the first part of your meditation.

Now, for the second part: Notice how you see yourself. Your qualities and how you feel, both today and in general. Are you tired today? Do you feel heavy, spacey, lazy? In general, do you see yourself as capable or stubborn or smart or funny? What are the words that jump into your mind when you contemplate how you see your-self?

Remember to be an observer. You are just trying to notice and not judge—so no commentary allowed.

Mind Makeover

Write down your defining characteristics. What are they

- in your body?
- at work?
- in your love and family relationships (as partner, spouse, lover, parent, sibling, child, friend)?

For each category, write down your strengths and your challenges. Try not to judge or filter—think of this as a brainstorming session, where there are no wrong answers. Be totally uninhibited.

Once you're finished, go back and review your characteristics. Notice whether you've listed more strengths or more challenges in some areas. Can you balance out the two lists a bit? They don't have to be perfectly equal, but try to get a nice symmetry between strengths and challenges. For example, if you're finding a lot of challenges in the physical category, think of some strengths—even if (especially if!) it feels difficult to do. You can always find something about your person that you like. Maybe it's your hair, your eyes, your forearms—any aspect of your body that, when you see it or feel it, you feel pride and happiness about. When it comes to work and relationships, are the two lists about equal—and if not, why not? Could how you perceive yourself in your relationships or at work be influencing your approach to self-care?

(After a couple of weeks on this retreat, you may find it helpful to review this list in order to recognize whether you've been saying things about yourself that you didn't even realize.)

....

TODAY'S MANTRA:

I am me.

....

Building Awareness

As you go through the rest of your day, remind yourself of the mantra and notice how those defining characteristics show up in your interactions and in your moments alone. As you're interacting at work, notice how the ways in which you see yourself affect how you interact with people. If you exercise, notice how the way you see yourself affects the way you move. Notice how the way you see yourself influences how you interact with your family or your loved ones.

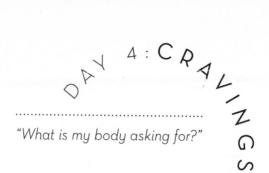

DAY 4: CRAVINGS

....

"What is my body asking for?"

In a world that constantly stimulates our senses, it's hard to resist so many triggers to satisfy our cravings. In any one day, our cravings can swing through hundreds of focal points: *I want that new pair of shoes. I wish I had a flatter stomach. What I would give for that dessert. I really want a glass of wine. How much longer till 5 p.m.?* Our minds are constantly searching for the next desire to chew on.

A big part of developing a meditation practice has to do with acknowledging that these thought streams and cravings are part of being human. But we also need to look beneath the surface to see what's driving them.

When it comes to weight loss, sugar is one of the

most difficult cravings to manage. It creates an endless cycle of wanting more. Besides tanking our blood sugar, driving up our cortisol, and trip-wiring our metabolism, sugar drives us to constantly look for our next fix. Have you ever felt satiated and content after a brownie? Most of us finish our dessert and start thinking about more. Whether we're on a diet or not, most don't feel calm or content after we eat sugar. We just want *moremoremore.*

I believe that it's healthy to give in to these cravings from time to time. But how do we find balance? Cravings fill a purpose, and unless we look at that purpose the cravings will never go away. Obviously, *what* we eat for the rest of the day is also very important, but our mental awareness of *why* we eat is also crucial to restructuring our metabolism (and often overlooked in diet plans and books).

Today I'd like you to consider the emotional purpose of these cravings. If it's sugar you're craving, reflect on what sort of sweetness you need in your life right now. Are you craving sweetness or affection from your partner? Are you craving more energy? Self-love? Are you craving attention, appreciation, connection, approval, stillness, less stress, less pressure, a vacation, time with your family, love from your children, love from your parents?

When you're hit with a craving, can you sit with it long enough to consider what's under it, even just for one minute? Just doing that—taking that one-minute pause—can honestly have the most profound effect on your health and your waistline. Can you broaden the gap between craving and filling your mouth (or buying new shoes or drinking that glass of wine)? Can you sit in the moment with the discomfort or sadness or guilt that lies underneath it?

Now, it's not my intention that you be swallowed up by emotions while meditating—though, if that happens, and you feel strong enough, go ahead and sit with them, let them lurk, and see what's there. My intention is that you become aware of those emotions, shine a light on them to see what's actually happening underneath your cravings. Once you do that, you have created another option for yourself:

> Do I eat the brownie, or do I talk to my partner?
> Do I hate the mirror, or do I take off my makeup for the day, appreciate my natural beauty, and love myself?
> Do I eat the chips, or go for food that will give me sustained energy?
> Do I eat it—or do I sit and meditate, even for just a few minutes, to consider what's happening

and what my body actually needs? Do I need
nourishment? Do I need to relax, connect,
sleep?
Can I find a way to answer that need from the
body in a way that leaves me feeling more
content?

The answer some days may be yes. Other days, no. There may be times when you're bonding with friends and enjoying food and being social and a craving strikes. In those times, is it appropriate to allow yourself to indulge? Or has that become a regular occurrence that could be affecting your health?

You'll find no wrong answers on day 4—this really is a personal process of reflection. Try not to judge yourself, and just watch what happens. Consider it an experiment—you are the study's subject, and you're trying to learn as much as you can about you.

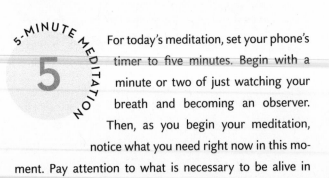

5-MINUTE MEDITATION

5

For today's meditation, set your phone's timer to five minutes. Begin with a minute or two of just watching your breath and becoming an observer. Then, as you begin your meditation, notice what you need right now in this moment. Pay attention to what is necessary to be alive in this moment. As you continue, notice how cravings come up in your meditation, things like wanting to move, or wanting to do things on your to-do list. As your to-do list comes up, you may start to think about all the things you need to do, and you may want to immediately jump up and do them! Notice whether you're hungry and craving certain foods, or maybe craving something like sleep or love or food or movement. See if you can notice those cravings and the feelings around them. Do you feel anxious or excited, happy or guilty? Are there any emotions attached to cravings? Then, even more important, notice the sensations that these thoughts create in your body. Notice what you feel and where you feel it. Notice if it feels uncomfortable to sit with these and not respond.

When the timer goes off, take a minute to finish by just watching the breath again.

When you're ready, open your eyes and grab your journal and pen.

Mind Makeover

Write about your cravings.

1. What are the foods or things that you crave on a regular basis? This could be a specific food (brownie) or a type of food

(sweets, crunchy, or salty food), or something like alcohol or caffeine, shopping, or checking your e-mail or social media.

2. Can you remember a time recently when you craved this thing? What do you think your body or spirit actually needed instead (time, less stress, attention, love, nutrients, energy, joy, compassion)?

3. How can you nourish that part of your body or soul today and feed that deep internal need (connecting with someone you love, eating more protein, getting more sleep)?

....

TODAY'S MANTRA:

What is my body asking for?

....

Building Awareness

As you go through your day, notice how many different cravings come up. When you notice one, consider what lies beneath it—what is your body/mind/spirit really asking for? Do this as often as you can today. How long you spend thinking about each one is not particularly important—it's more about noticing how often these cravings kick in and if there's a common theme behind them.

Remember, you're not concerned about doing everything perfectly. If you give in to a craving here or there, it isn't the end of the world. The purpose is to become more aware of what is *triggering* the cravings, so you can feed your body what it actually needs instead—whether that means food, fun, intimate connection, or compassion for yourself.

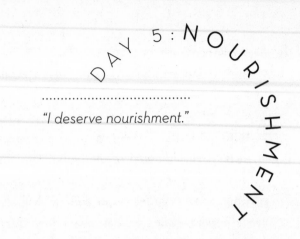

DAY 5: NOURISHMENT

"I deserve nourishment."

Today is about nourishment. We'll look at how our need for nourishment shows up not only in ourselves but also how it impacts our partners, spouses, kids, even our siblings, parents, and friends.

Many of us spend a lot of our time helping the people around us—and forgetting about ourselves or deliberately ignoring the things we want or need. We don't leave time for our own happiness and health. We find it much easier to focus on others, but we forget a very important point: Our health really *does* affect everyone around us. Turns out we really *do* have to put the proverbial oxygen mask on first before we can help the other passengers. In our rush to help loved ones, it's easy to forget to love ourselves. We forget how important our own nourishment is in protecting our ability to do just that.

I see patients all day long, and I do a lot of international travel to train teachers around the world. I know all too well how easy it is to get caught up in busy days and leave myself for last. But self-nourishment is so important, especially in a service industry. Seeing patients and training teachers creates a constant reminder for me that I have to come back, give back, to myself. I can be of service, but I can't give to anyone else unless I continue to take care of myself. That's the foundation of me being able to do my work.

I have a friend who used to make smoothies for her kids. She'd pack them with fresh and frozen fruits, high-quality yogurt, and omega-3s, and pour large glasses for her two girls. Then she'd go back and scrape out the blender with a spatula, dribbling out the remainder for herself. She basically took whatever was left.

One day she had a revelation: She could put out three glasses instead of two.

When I asked her why she had never thought of that before, she said, "I was always proud to serve them these super-healthy smoothies, dense with nutrition. But I just wasn't thinking of myself." It was really silly, and 100 percent subconscious. She was pouring everything she had into her kids and sustaining herself on their leavings. That moment of awareness stuck and helps her recognize when she has those limiting thoughts in other parts of her life, and when she needs to nourish herself instead.

Today is about making time to nourish ourselves, and noticing how our health really affects those around us.

We often think of our nourishment as strictly food-based, but our bodies have to be nourished on many levels, in many different ways. So many of our struggles with weight loss come from being malnourished—the body is holding on to fat or calories because it's not getting what it needs.

Today we will start to develop an awareness that nourishment comes in many forms. Yes, food is nourishment. But nourishment can also come in the form of love, laughter, and joy, in our connections to the people around us, in painting or gardening or reading, in attending the-ater or live music, or in the pursuit of good work. Sleep is a form of nourishment, our body's time to heal and repair and to process all the food we've taken in. We are nourished by sunlight and exercise and quiet. Fresh air nourishes us with oxygen from each breath.

We open our meditation today by focusing on what we think of as nourishment. As you come into meditation for these 5 minutes, after you have settled in, observe the quality of the breath—but today from a different stance, noticing that the breath is a form of nourishment. Think of the built-in transportation system that carries oxygen into every cell as a source of nourishment. Pay attention to how the breath comes into the body, and then follow it. Notice how it moves through the lungs, but also create an awareness of the breath really nourishing every cell of the body, out to the fingertips and the toes and the top of the head.

Mind Makeover

Today we consider nourishment.

1. How do you take time daily to nourish yourself? With food, air, love, downtime? Aside from food, what makes you feel nourished?

2. How does that nourishment affect your

work? Your family life and love life? Your health? Try to expand your thinking past the moment to later today, next month, and a year from now. Then ten years from now. What are the specific long-term effects that these types of nourishment will have on the other parts of your life? The more specific you can be, the more helpful it will be. Rather than *Taking time to nourish myself will improve my relationship,* dig a little deeper: *My ability to take time to nourish myself will allow me to connect more deeply and communicate more effectively with my partner and protect the longevity of our relationship.* Or *These potato chips might taste good right now. But eating potato chips for the next ten years will potentially shorten my life, widen my hips, and actually not nourish me in any way I'd truly like.*

3. Do you deserve to be healthy? How does your health affect the people around you— your children, parents, siblings, partner, or friends? How can you be a good example to your children so that they can find the same health and well-being in their lives?

4. We looked at presence on day 2. Have you noticed that your ability to be present with someone helps you connect with that person more deeply? How does that nourish you? If you can have that sense of depth in your connections, can you instill that in your loved ones or your kids? How will that change their lives?

....

TODAY'S MANTRA:
I deserve nourishment.

....

Building Awareness

As you go forward through your day, notice whether you believe that you deserve to be healthy. How does that thought show up during your day? If you find it difficult to agree with this mantra, as many women are surprised to discover that they do, why do you think that is? What is standing in the way of your total agreement? If you believe that you deserve to be healthy, what are the implications? How will you take care of yourself? What will you do differently?

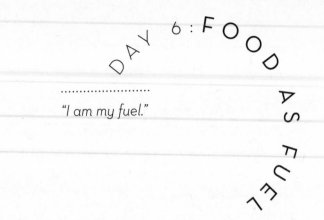

DAY 6: FOOD AS FUEL

....

"I am my fuel."

Yesterday we looked at nourishing ourselves with things other than food. Today we'll think about food itself. Now that you've shifted your mind-set about nourishment to all of those things that truly feed you, let's consider how we think about food and try to shift our perspective from seeing food as calories, as "fattening" or "diet food," and instead see it as a source of nourishment.

Of all the diets out there, one of the most limiting is old-school calorie counting. When I'm working with a patient who is trying to lose weight, one of the first things I often do is have her stop counting calories. Surprised? We sometimes get so perfectionistic about the math, we can forget that what's actually *in* our foods can vary dramatically. Even among foods with the same number of calories, the nutrition level can vary dramatically. We can eat the "correct" number of calories or points or servings but still be eating mostly nutritionally bankrupt foods.

One of my patients, Gail, used to write down every single food she ate every day, counting her calories to a tee, so she knew exactly how many calories she had consumed or would consume at any time. She brought a three-ring binder filled with many months of her food journals to our first appointment.

Right away, I could see that the calorie counting had become a compulsion for Gail, a way of managing her hopes and fears about her weight, so I didn't ask her to go cold turkey. Instead, I started planting seeds. I asked her to do some short meditations about how she feeds the machine of her body, not only with calories but with nutrients. She thought about questions such as *What is it that I'm putting in my body? How is it feeding this machine? What does my body actually need?*

She continued to count and record her calories, but as her awareness grew through meditation, she started to see clear distinctions between her foods— not just in the calories but in how she felt after eating different food combinations. Eventually, she gravitated away from the journaling as she started to refer to what I like to call the owner's manual to her body; she was able to listen and observe what worked for her, without external cues (including compulsive calorie counting).

Despite more than a year of slavish devotion to her journal, Gail's weight had not budged. But once she started meditating, something shifted, and the weight started to come off.

Eventually, she lost the twenty pounds she was aiming for, and we worked together until she felt she could sustain her health on her own. When I saw her a year later, she looked as if she'd lost a few more pounds. But even more important, she looked healthy and happy—the most desirable outcome, and the least quantifiable.

When we're doing something difficult or scary, we can put a lot of stock into outside guidance, looking for a metric to tell us we're "doing it right." We want scales. We want calories. We want pounds.

But all of these numbers are relative. Any woman can tell you that weight often fluctuates from one day to the next by several pounds, just based on water weight—especially on days with extra hormonal flux. How wonderful would it be if we could get away from that "how to lose 5 pounds in 5 days" or "how to lose 15 pounds in 1 month" mentality? When we shift our focus from losing weight to gaining health, we can still let go of extra pounds—but we also gain so much more in the process.

Your body is a machine, and food is how you fuel the machine. Thinking about your body as a machine might seem cold—but what if we thought of food as purely fuel? Separate from our mind-body connection, separate from any emotional attachment or cravings. What if we could simply say, *Yes, my body is a machine. And if I pour sludge into it, it's going to run a little slower. But if I feed it and nourish it with high-octane fuel, it's going to help the whole system.*

You would never expect a car to run on water (or sugar!) instead of gas. Why are you depriving yourself in the name of better health? Why is it that we feel the need to deprive ourselves to be healthy? And what happens when we switch our mind-set from deprivation to feeding ourselves to thrive?

You're shifting away from weight loss and toward health. You're shifting away from calories and toward the right balance of protein, fats, and carbs for your unique constitution. (Check out chapter 6 for eating guidelines and a food map.) Each of those nutrients, each vitamin and mineral, fuels a different process in your body. Those nutrients are required for different metabolic components—not just the "metabolism" we think about in terms of weight loss but also the body's ability to process everything it needs.

If you get nothing else out of this book, I would like you to stop thinking about calories and start to change your mind-set from losing weight to nourishing the body. Food helps you optimize your body's functions, including its ability to metabolize food! Changing your focus from weight loss to nourishing yourself is a way to create real, lasting change in your relationship with food.

As you settle yourself for meditation, notice the body as a machine. Just be aware of what's happening inside the container of your body, studying the inner workings.

This meditation has three steps, working from large-scale to more subtle refinements. The first part is just noticing the more obvious sensations, such as heart rate and the breath. Next, I want you to notice the circulation and temperature of your body. Finally, notice the more subtle current of energy under the skin.

Energy is a hard thing to define, to prove or disprove. In Chinese medicine, one of my favorite definitions of *qi* is "energy on the verge of materializing." Your qi is the potential underneath your skin to do, to move, to create, to exercise, to hold your kids—before it actually takes place. Notice that very subtle current of potential that pulsates right underneath the skin. Notice the sense of energy in the body and its connection to the life of the body in its more large-scale forms: the heart, the breath, the circulation and temperature.

In this meditation you'll just sit and notice the inner container of the body, the machine that enables you to sit and watch and notice the gross and subtle sensations in the heart, breath, circulation, temperature, and energy as well as any other sensations you become aware of. Notice this experience of life in the body. Find the awe in this life that we all have, and in our ability to notice it.

Mind Makeover

Today our journaling will connect with the work of day 5.

1. Recall the foods you ate yesterday. Write down everything you can remember eating.

2. Reflect on what caused you to eat each food or meal. How might you choose differently if you were emotionally detached?

3. Plan your fuel for the next 24 hours, in as much detail as you can. Consider what raw materials you have in the kitchen, and which restaurants or takeout spots are available to you. Your plan doesn't need to be perfect—this is an experiment. You are just noticing how you can best plan your fuel based on what you have to work with.

....
TODAY'S MANTRA:
I am my fuel.
....

Building Awareness

As you go through your day, take a moment to remember the day's mantra and see how the image of being your own fuel shows up in your interactions and in your moments alone. What does this mantra mean to you?

From your journal, copy out your plan for your breakfast, morning and afternoon snacks, lunch, and dinner for today (or tomorrow, if completing this at night). Set a timer around 10 a.m. and 3 p.m., and plan to have your snacks then. When you're done eating your snack, review your plan for lunch. Do the same thing in the afternoon, with your snack and your dinner. Snacks help you fuel the body but also prevent you from getting into a position where hunger drives you and the emotions start taking over. Healthy snacks ward off the craving for carbs for instant fuel—the breads, pastas, sandwiches—and the emotional attachment to those cravings. And you'll be better able to feed your machine before it starts sputtering and you get that desperate, clingy, needy feeling. Making a plan and checking in with yourself during the day will help you separate the cravings of the emotional body from the physical body's need for fuel.

Notice how you feel throughout the day today, especially before and after meals. How is your fuel serving you? Are you able to think about eating in advance of being ravenously hungry? Try this as you're sitting in a restaurant, considering the menu. Or maybe when you're in a meeting and you find yourself thinking about food. One of the biggest things I want you to pay attention to is how you feel *before* you get hungry.

Eating well to fuel yourself can be really difficult. We can get emotionally attached to hunger as soon as we start to feel it. We start to crave certain things. Notice how being able to plan your fuel ahead and consider your feelings and fuel beforehand can have an impact on how you manage your eating.

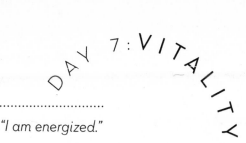

DAY 7: VITALITY

....

"I am energized."

Today is all about the importance of your energy level.

We need energy for many things—for our work, our family, our self-care. We need to have enough energy left for ourselves and our partners at the end of the day, to be able to nourish our relationships. But there's also one often forgotten or neglected but crucial aspect of energy management: having the energy to be able to have fun and relax and enjoy our lives. We need to be efficient enough in our work and in meeting our obligations that we have time and energy left for the parts of life that make it truly worth living.

Many of us go through our days and just write off

feelings of lethargy and fatigue as normal. But can we reconsider and determine if that's truly accurate? What if that wasn't our reality? What if our energy level were different? What if we didn't have those lulls?

These past few days, we've been thinking a lot about how we nourish ourselves to protect our energy levels. Then we talked about the frequency of our meals—fueling the machine before the emotional body gets involved. Today we'll talk a little bit about our body's digestive process—our ability to extract exactly what we need from our foods.

Energy level is one way to quickly get a sense of whether or not you're feeding your machine the right things. The energy changes caused by what you eat don't necessarily come immediately after you eat. You might not get these signals for several hours. Your afternoon lull could be connected with the quality of the fuel you've eaten for breakfast or lunch. And food is not the only thing that affects our energy levels; many other aspects of nourishment—sleep, air, water, healthy relationships, rewarding work—have a great influence. But for now, let's look closely at food, and our digestion, through energy.

Yesterday we talked about tuning in to our internal signals and getting ahead of our gnawing hunger. The truth is, the optimal frequency of meals really depends on our individual digestion. Some who digest quickly really need to eat every few hours. Those who digest more slowly may need more time between meals. Digestion is another aspect of our health where we can place our attention, separating *what my mouth wants* and *what my emotional body wants* from *the signals I am feeling in my stomach or my energy level.*

Most of us know what it feels like to have that gnawing, empty feeling in the stomach, when we're *really* hungry, versus the experience of the mind and mouth wanting something while our stomachs still feel full. We may have just finished a big dinner, but we still crave dessert. We can begin to use our awareness to work on our ability to separate those feelings. When we learn to notice how quickly we digest our food, we are better able to gauge how frequently we should be eating—and how much.

As you pay closer attention to these signals, you'll likely notice that the most sustainable fuel comes from the right ratios of fats, fiber, and protein. Fats trigger the satiety reflex in the stomach, helping our bodies feel satisfied. Fiber and protein take longer for the stomach to process than refined carbohydrate, slowing down the release of glucose into our blood, so they'll give us more sustainable fuel throughout the day.

When you consider your meals, either those yesterday or those you plan to eat in the next 24 hours, notice when you have more fats, proteins, and fiber-rich foods. Notice how those foods affect your experience of your blood sugar—do they sustain you longer? Despite carbs being demonized, we do still need them—they are important brain food, helping us think and function well—but how do different carbs affect your energy level? How soon do you feel hungry after eating a meal of simple carbs like pasta compared with one containing whole grains and protein? Pay attention, observe, create that awareness in your body.

For people who tend to get very tired during the day, I have found one of two common scenarios to be true: they are eating too much—they go to lunch, eat a lot, come back, and fall into an afternoon haze—or they are not eating often enough—skipping breakfast or a morning snack and not eating anything until 1 p.m. By the time they actually get food into their system, their bodies are in recovery mode, making it difficult for their blood sugar to balance out. Notice if one of those scenarios resonates with you.

Now let's consider how your body processes that food. Digestion is key. If you're not digesting well, you may experience indigestion or irregular bowel movements. Indigestion—signaled by excess gas, intestinal pain, or heartburn—is a signal that the body is not extracting the vital nutrients from the food you eat (even very good food). Of course, please check out any bothersome digestive complaints with your health care practitioner (which could be your primary care doctor, or your naturopath or acupuncturist—someone you trust). But if you've done that and you're still struggling, there's something we can all do to help our bodies every day: slow down.

Allowing our natural digestive system the time to fully execute its processes will help our body to better absorb nutrients. This process starts from the moment we begin to cook—we start to smell the food, which triggers salivation and the release of acid in the stomach, preparing the body to digest the food more efficiently. Then the process of slowly chewing our food physically breaks it down and mixes it with the enzymes in the saliva, preparing the body for further breakdown of food in the stomach. We benefit at each of these points along the chain when we can remind ourselves to slow down and savor our food.

Slowing down also helps the nervous system component. As we start to slow down, the parasympathetic nervous system kicks in, which triggers our rest-and-digest response. In contrast, when we charge through our meals and eat our food really quickly, we trigger the sympathetic nervous system—especially when we're stressed and thinking and we've got our eyes on our computer, mindlessly stuffing food in our mouths. Our sympathetic nervous system isn't prepared to digest the food—so digestion is interrupted, rerouted, taken out of its natural flow and rhythm, often causing indigestion or other intestinal upset and poor absorption of the nutrients critical for energy.

Both the content of what we eat and the manner in which we eat can really affect our digestion. You can eat all the right things and still not feel good if the body is not digesting properly—and that is when we start to crave. Cravings are often the body telling us that it needs something—but in order to understand what's behind those cravings, instead of simply reacting and eating whatever our body is craving, we must slow down and listen. That's what today's meditation is all about.

Today, for the first minute or two, settle into your breathing and your observer stance. Notice your energy level today and how it affects your posture and your mood.

Then, as you're noticing the breath, I want you to visualize taking in energy. Visualize your breath as pure energy coming into the cells, oxygenating the cells; see it as the fuel that drives the cellular process that creates energy in our bodies. Then, on each exhale, visualize letting go of fatigue, dullness, or anything that weighs you down mentally or physically.

Remember: Rather than trying to actually deepen or control the breath, you're just watching the natural pace of the breath; this isn't a breathing exercise. As you inhale each time, you're visualizing energy coming in naturally and just acknowledging that energy comes in through the breath into your body to invigorate you. And then as you exhale, you're letting go of anything that weighs you down.

Do this for a few minutes, then drop back to just noticing and observing the experience of your breath in your body. If you enjoy this and lose track of time don't worry, you can do it for the entire 5 minutes if you like— whatever feels comfortable to you. When you reach the end of the meditation, once your timer goes off, take a moment with your eyes still closed, just to notice the change in your energy level and how your body feels.

Mind Makeover

Today you'll journal about your energy and vitality.

1. Write down what you ate yesterday, and note any dips in your energy during the day.
2. Based on the past few days' experience, what have you learned about your habits, and how can they inform today's eating? Write down a general meal plan for the day.
3. Decide on a few specific moments today when you will check in with your energy, and write them down.

TODAY'S MANTRA:
I am energized.

Building Awareness

As you go through your day, recall your mantra, noticing any changes in energy as an extension of what and how you eat, so you can start to construct your own food map. Study yourself as if in an experiment. How do you feel when you eat certain foods? Does your fatigue limit you? Remember that sometimes cravings are our bodies telling us they need something nutritionally different. Also recall that by doing simple things, such as chewing better and slowing down during meals, we can increase absorption of nutrients and indirectly increase energy and decrease cravings.

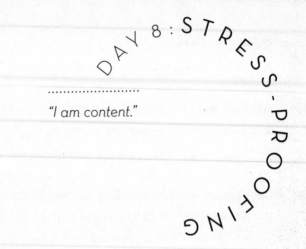

....

"I am content."

Meditation is based on the idea that it's not the stressor itself that's the issue but our reaction to it and our judgment of it that matters. When we learn to detach from our perception of stress the same way we observe the breath in meditation, when we learn to tell ourselves, *I am okay; this too shall pass,* without getting involved in our worries, we can block the negative effects of stress on our bodies, both physiologically and mentally.

My patient Lisa was a classic type A, stressed-out person. She ate pretty well and exercised a little bit— which was a great start, considering her demanding 60-hour workweeks. But you could see the stress on her face when she would come in for treatments. She had a hard time lying still on the table. She always had her phone switched on—even during our acupuncture sessions. Clearly her biggest issue was stress—but very soon after we added meditation to her program, she effortlessly lost twenty pounds. She noticed her efficiency at work improving, which allowed her more time for herself, and her stress level was much lower. She looked and felt so much happier, and her metabolism just sorted itself out naturally. All simply from adding meditation.

If we're not careful, even a healthy "stress" such as endurance exercise and training can turn into a negative stress—especially when we overestimate what our system can handle. A few years ago I was treating Amy, a runner. She ran two marathons a year, in addition to being the mother of two and working a full-time job. She had a very healthy, balanced diet. But she was still about twenty pounds heavier than what was healthy for her body, and I suspected it had a lot to do with the messages her lifestyle was sending to her body: *I am under constant stress.*

With Amy, all we had to do was *decrease* her running a bit, and add in 10 minutes a day of meditation—and she ended up losing ten pounds in less than eight weeks. What Amy needed was to help her body shift into parasympathetic mode a bit more often every day.

Just having two kids can be a full-time job, but add a demanding career and a high-mileage running regimen, and anyone's body is bound to say uncle. I like to tell this story because I find that everyone thinks "more exercise = weight loss." But sometimes exercising less and meditating more is the best solution.

Today I'd like you to recognize how great an effect stress has on both your brain function and your metabolism. We all feel overwhelmed at times, getting caught up in the drama of the moment, but when we look back just a few months later, the precipitating event seems so small and insignificant. Being able to consistently keep the big picture in view is a gift to our metabolism—and to our sanity.

Stress is really your body's response to your *interpretation* of what's happening, your own personal version of reality, and it is totally relative to each person. You could be shouldering the same amount of responsibility as someone else—yet he might feel stress and you might not. Stress is really just a by-product of our interpretation of our experience.

In this meditation practice, we're trying to use an observer's mind-set to broaden the gap between a trigger and our response. When we're in a stressful situation, we can learn to pause for a moment to just notice our reaction, before we yell or panic or internalize the stress. That pause might help us change how we react to another person, which could change the dynamic of the entire situation.

And when we do make a shift, it doesn't need to be worlds away from where we already are. You might yell out a four-letter word cluster at the office or at home. You might have an argument with your mother or your spouse. If you're able to notice your reaction, you can breathe and cut back the stress reactivity of your internal experience, shorten your own fight-or-flight response, and thereby decrease your cortisol. These changes can make an immediate difference in how you communicate with your partner as well as how you experience that moment in your body.

There's something liberating about realizing that you don't have to orchestrate monumental changes to better manage internal conflict, and that incremental changes really do work. You don't have to be perfect—either in physicality or in thought.

Today's meditation is all about developing your ability to notice the sensations in each breath but then also see the bigger picture. The first part is to observe the breath and acknowledge the sensations in the body and see if you can detangle them from the mind. Then recount a stressful situation or a stressful day—anything recent enough that you can recall it in full detail and really connect to that memory. Notice the sensations that the recollection brings up in the body. Is it possible to allow the sensations to exist and to disengage the mind, to just notice and watch them? Take a moment to do this. Then notice what it feels like to acknowledge that everything will pass at some point. Consider that in the big picture, a month or a year from now, you'll look back on this one little stressful experience and it will be insignificant. Last, notice what it feels like to acknowledge that right now, in this moment, you have everything you need.

Mind Makeover

Today's journaling will focus on stressful moments.

1. Notice your stress points, either from yesterday or last week, whether they're minor incidents, ongoing situations, or big events.
2. Ask yourself, how different would those stress points look if you were able to take

an observer's mind-set? To detach your-self in the moment when you feel stress and simply observe? Notice the experi-ence and imagine the big picture.

3. Will the outcome of those moments look different? Sometimes it will, and some-times it won't. How will it be different? Remember, today's work is not necessar-ily changing stress or outcomes but rather changing your perception. That shift alone has a profound effect on your health.

TODAY'S MANTRA:
I am content.

Building Awareness

Today, as an experiment, notice your stress levels and how your perceptions can change the outcome of a situation, whether it's for yourself or others. Rather than obsessing or worrying about a dreaded project, is it possible to be efficient and just get things done, and be able to enjoy the process? Notice the impact of your stress levels on the situation itself—does stress make you more or less efficient? Does it improve or harm your interactions with others? Does it impact your personal health and your sense of comfort in yourself?

If you tend toward overwork (or use other forms of excessive compensation), ask yourself as you go along today if you feel unworthy unless you work to the extreme—is there a psychological backdrop at work here? Is there some element of you thriving on that busyness and that stress?

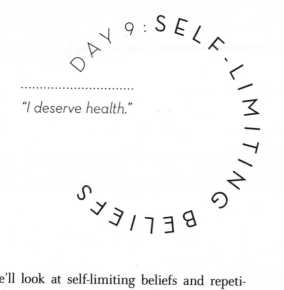

DAY 9: SELF-LIMITING BELIEFS

....

"I deserve health."

Today we'll look at self-limiting beliefs and repetitive, destructive self-analysis. What do you subconsciously tell yourself about your worth on a daily basis? Now we'll question if it's true. *(Am I worthless? Am I instead good enough? Do I believe I deserve to be healthy? To be vibrant? To be my best self?)* How you see your worth in the world and what you have to contribute is a key to lightening up in all senses of the word.

I grew up working in a homeless shelter run by my mom. One thing that I saw over and over among this population was a sense of low expectations. Partly, this feeling was in the residents themselves, but I grew to realize that no one ever really expected them to succeed or believed in them.

We provided food and shelter, but most of what we did was provide a support system for them so they could start to believe in themselves. Some of that was through getting them the education or job skills they needed. But I think there was also a subconscious level in supporting them and believing in them when they had no one else who did. We expected things of them and held them accountable.

We all have a part of us that is motivated by the expectations of the people around us. We all have expectations that were imposed on us by our families, friends, and colleagues, and the people around us—but also by ourselves. These expectations can either lift us up or push us down—and both types affect how and whether we achieve our goals, whether in work or in weight loss. If we internalize negative expectations, our own lowered expectations and self-limiting beliefs will become destructive not only to our minds but also to our bodies.

The secret to overcoming self-limiting expectations that root down into beliefs is simply becoming conscious of them. I liken it to going into your closet to pick out clothes with the lights off and hoping you come out with something that works—versus going in and turning on the light and deciding. You might leave behind the shirt that's all beat up or you might wear it, but you can at least make a conscious decision about what you are choosing to wear for the day. And just as with clothing, what thoughts and beliefs you choose to hold are not right or wrong—you simply want to see which ones you're allowing into your head.

What's interesting is how these expectations can show up in our work, the way we pursue our goals, how we interact with our friends, and what we expect of our kids and our partners. This is, as we become more conscious of it, where we get the opportunity to begin to rewrite our story. We can look and see and ask ourselves, *Is this accurate? Am I expecting too much of myself? Am I expecting too little?*

We have to begin to notice how our expectations create our life and how we approach tasks. We need to watch basic, easy-to-identify things, like how we approach a project that's overwhelming versus how we approach a task that's easy. We'll then see how our expectations change our approach. If we have a task that seems overwhelming, but we can interpret it in a different way, we might be able to process it differently. Remember our work from yesterday: Our nervous system processes everything based on our perspective.

I love to play with this idea in my yoga teacher training classes. At some point, some pictures of me doing fancy poses got around, so now I'm seen as someone who likes to do fancy poses. One thing I absolutely love to do is not so much the poses themselves but to sneak people into them. Yoga is very interesting in that you can really break it down step by step. If I can walk people though the process step by step, they often surprise themselves in their ability to do something that seems at first overwhelming and impossible. Often when I do demonstrations, a majority of the room actually ends up getting into the pose that previously seemed so unattainable. It's not a magic trick; it's not like I wave a wand and all of a sudden they're able to do it. What makes it possible is their capacity to believe in their potential and get out of their own way in getting there.

In our lives we have to be able to visualize that potential as well. For our nervous system to see anything through to completion—whether it's a task at work or a yoga pose—our mind has to be able to conceive of its possibility. So today, one of the big things I would like us to notice is the ways we block our own growth and success.

When it comes to our mental health, our self-concept plays a really large role. Nowadays, even the layperson knows how much our mental health is linked to physical health, how much they interact and depend upon each other. The media surrounds us with reminders of the ways in which we are not measuring up to the healthy ideal, the ways we need to be more and do more. Those messages can leave us feeling worthless. And when we don't live up to what we expect of ourselves, or to what we want, our disappointment in ourselves also can leave us feeling worthless.

I was teased a lot as a kid, and I learned really quickly how to be strong and to create my life—I became a strong yoga teacher and medical practitioner. I educated myself really well. At one point I noticed that I still felt this underlying need for approval; I abused myself by overworking, feeling like I had to be more or do more. I was functioning from a sense of lack rather than a sense of abundance.

In my experience, healing is not so much about getting rid of that feeling. I can't go back to when I was taunted as a kid and change that. Those experiences teach us to grow in different ways; they form and develop us. They can, in that way, be very valuable. Yet if we continue to function from that sense of lack, it negatively affects the way we approach our-selves and our world.

Just being able to acknowledge where a feeling came from and see how it is expressed in our lives grants us the ability to let it go, just as a kid who can summon the courage to look under the bed realizes that there is no monster. If I can just see where the feeling of being less than is coming from, if I can look it in the eye, then I may see that it's not really scary for me anymore. I can see how these things helped shape me in the past and how they affect how I inter-act now. I don't need to get rid of them—I just need to be able to acknowledge them.

Today is about getting clear, looking at how ex-pectations, high or low, can affect us—by preventing us from believing in ourselves or by setting us up for failure.

Settle into your favorite meditation spot and begin to notice your breath-ing. As you close your eyes tune in to the inner landscape of your body and notice how you feel today mentally and emotionally. Notice if there is any prominent negative talk going on in the background of your mind as your mind sits with the content from this chapter.

Begin to tune in to that self-talk and pick out one of those toxic emotions, whatever is most prominent for you right now—whether it's stress or anger or feeling worthless, or not being able to live up to expectations, or not feeling good enough, or feeling overwhelmed. Just pick one toxic mind-set that feels the most prominent to you today.

While you are sitting, breathe naturally. Notice what this toxic emotion feels like. Notice the quality and the sensations of that feeling. Where do you experience these sensations in your body? What part of your body? What's the quality of it; is it heavy or thick or dark? Notice your ability to visualize those feelings, and gather that emotional experience. Each time you inhale, imagine your breath gathering the accumulation of that toxic emotion into one spot in your body. Then, on the exhale—let it go.

Repeat that same process for the entire 5 minutes of meditation. Just imagine those feelings consolidating and getting smaller and smaller, gathering into a more condensed area—until you can release it all.

Mind Makeover

Today's writing will focus on noticing how your expectations and your beliefs shape your interactions with important aspects of your life. For each of the following, quickly write down your beliefs about yourself and your expectations. Then note how those beliefs have impacted each area.

1. Your work and your goals.
2. Your family and your partner or loved one.
3. Your hobbies, exercise, yoga practice, or other similar activity or passion.
4. Most important, your belief in what you are able to accomplish in this lifetime.

....

TODAY'S MANTRA:
I deserve health.

....

Building Awareness

As you go through the day, remind yourself of the mantra and notice how the defining characteristics of health show up in your interactions and in your moments alone. Consider again the question: Do I believe I deserve to be healthy? In every sense—mind, body, and spirit?

Throughout the day, take time to further reflect on your journal responses, and add to them as new thoughts come to you.

DAY 10: RADIANCE

....

"I am healthy."

On day 10 we're going to simplify things.

When we think about being healthy, we often think about having to take more supplements or eat less or exercise more. Instead, today I want us to look at health as something that already exists inside of each one of us.

Our bodies evolved with many checks and balances built in, with many ways that the body can heal and repair itself. We have a natural state of health that exists underneath it all that often gets covered up. The older we get, the more time we've had to cover that up, the further buried that innate health may be.

I believe that this burying effect accounts for

much of what we view as the aging process, over time, with one lifestyle choice after another. Consider plants: We don't talk about plants as being old. But if you took two plants and poured Coca-Cola on one and fresh water on the other, the appearance and the health of the two plants would be very different.

Obviously our physiology undergoes some degeneration over time, on a much larger scale. But I think a big part of what we see as we get older is that we have longer to collect the toxins we pour into our bodies, physically and mentally. These inputs and experiences go into forming our health. Achieving radiant health can simply be a matter of countering the effects of that buildup to uncover what's already there.

One of the core principles in Chinese medicine, including acupuncture and its reliance on the meridians, is that our bodies know how to heal themselves. Energetic channels, or meridians, run through every part of the body. Just like the rivers that once transported food and supplies from one village or city to another, the meridians are thought to be tributaries that encourage the transport of nutrients, energy, and blood supply throughout the body. Acupuncture holds that blockages occur when our bodies have a hard time healing and repairing because they can't get the nutrients and supplies they need. We need certain nutrients to be able to perform specific functions, and if our bodies are not able to receive those nutrients, we can't heal, and we can't achieve homeostasis. But if we can remove the sludge that's clogging up our system, eliminate the obstacles that stand in our way and the burdens that weigh us down, we can rebalance the body and uncover our health.

Over the past ten days we've looked at what foods we eat and how we eat them. We've looked at stress— how much we have and how we approach it. When we think about what else is loading up in our bodies, we may realize we simply have too much on our plates, both literal and metaphorical: too many menial tasks, too much to do as a parent, too much worrying about work, too much of eating the wrong foods.

As we look at the things that weigh us down and how we can uncover our health and our body's ability to heal, we also have to look at our body's ability to process what it's given. Consider the liver and its detox pathways, for instance. The liver can process only a certain amount of substances, and once its detox pathways start to clog up, the remaining toxins just sit in the body, getting stored in the tissues and the cells. This load on the body can come from foods, or it can come from pharmaceuticals, toxins from the air and water, hormonal imbalances—it can even come from a lack of social connection or an unfulfilling job. The combination of all these factors determines how much burden the body is able to process at any given time.

We have to start to look at what we can take off this list. What's reasonable? What can you remove from your body's processing system? What's weighing you down? As you remove the sludge, health becomes something to *uncover* rather than something to *accomplish*. It's already there, a buried treasure waiting to sparkle.

More than two decades ago, when I first trained to be a teacher, I remember hearing about the idea of enlightenment, which we Westerners don't really think about so much. The concept can seem really intimidating and overwhelming. But what fascinated me was the way it was spoken of as something that already exists, in each of us, something that we just have to wake up to and uncover.

To me, in our modern world, the manifestation of this enlightenment is our ability to consciously connect and be present in our lives, and that encompasses being present to our own capacity for beautiful, radiant health. Our good health already exists. We just have to uncover it.

In today's meditation I want you to connect with the sense of health that already exists inside of you. Begin by sitting and noticing what's happening inside of your body today. See if you can put your finger on the quality of health inside your body and notice exactly what it feels like. Is it a specific or a general feeling? Does your brain go to work to try to analyze this, or can you just see what your experience is in your body today without judgment or predicting? Notice if there's a part of you that can connect and actually visualize a sense of health on a cellular basis.

You might notice this feeling of health in one part of your body more than another. You might have a more difficult time experiencing it in certain parts of your body. Whether you're injured or ill or sick, it doesn't really matter why. You don't need to really analyze it. Instead notice your ability to visualize a sense of health as something that really does exist in you—something that's already there.

Mind Makeover

Notice the sense of health that already exists within you.

1. After doing the visualization and really acknowledging that there is a sense of health inside of you, how will you choose your foods differently?

2. How will you interact with yourself and others differently? Sometimes getting to a place where you feel good again can be very difficult. But once you do feel good, it's harder to pour toxic things into your body. Once you can visualize your innate health, you will have a new perspective on what your body wants and deserves.

....

TODAY'S MANTRA:
I am healthy.

....

Building Awareness

As you go through your day, ask yourself, *What do I actually need?* Consider this in relation to your food:

How little or how much do I need to sustain myself and feel good? Or in relation to your work: *What do I actually need to do today to be efficient?* Or in your relationships: *What do I need to do to connect with the people in my life in a way that feeds me?*

Once you recognize what you truly *need* today, allow yourself to let go of the rest. Let go of the menial tasks and the mindless distractions and all the garbage that you always feel like you have to do. Today, just look at what you *need*.

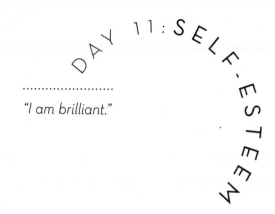

....

"I am brilliant."

We talk a lot about intelligence. We talk a lot about Alzheimer's disease and the state of our brains, about staying smart and mentally fit. But I'd like us to question this view of intelligence and shift it a bit.

Your intelligence is not dictated by your IQ specifically, or how stereotypically "smart" you are. Your intelligence also encompasses how you contribute to the world. Your contributions, whatever they may be, are the mark that you make and the offering that you give back to the world.

I believe that each of us is born with a purpose. We all have specific, unique gifts, and we have a responsibility to give our gifts to the world. As a community, both small and large, we have to really understand those strengths to function well. Measuring our intelligence exclusively in IQ points is not going to help us as a community, as a globe, as a family, let alone individually. Our contribution and unique gifts are really our intelligence.

Think about the trash collector versus the president. Many kids say they want to be president. How many times did you hear that in your grade school? But kids rarely say, *When I grow up, I want to be the trash collector.* But if we didn't have someone collecting trash, this would be a pretty horrible, ugly place to live. The job of the trash collector is just as significant as that of president. Understanding that our contribution is uniquely significant is crucial to our health.

The other thing we'll be thinking about today is knowledge: our innate knowledge or wisdom regarding our health. Often we block this knowledge with conscious thought by trying to figure out the perfect diet or the perfect meal plan, instead of asking, *What does my body need?* and really listening. Our bodies know what we need.

The hard thing is distinguishing this internal knowledge of need from the emotion of craving. Being able to look as an observer helps us to see what is emotional attachment and what is simply your body saying, *Yes, you actually probably need to eat now.* The more you adopt an observer's stance, the more information your body will give you.

We don't need to read all the right nutrition books or even to find the right diet to achieve health; all we need to do is observe how our bodies respond— whether to food or to our mental state, as we've discussed over the past week or so.

Reshape your perception around what genius is. For me, genius might be understanding certain yoga poses so that I can help my patients better. For the president, genius might be being able to make tough decisions and leading people through hard times and change. Our genius is in our unique contribution.

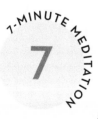

In today's meditation, you'll come back to the observer's mind-set. This time you're bringing your awareness to the palms of your hands. Start by noticing and becoming aware of the sensation in the palms of your hands. You may notice things like warmth or circulation, or a sense of more subtle energy. You don't need to put words to it, just notice.

And then pay attention to that sense of the potential in your palms and in your fingertips as an extension of your capability and potential. Notice your intelligence as a combination of your mind and body, coordinated by your unique purpose on this planet. Consider the potential at your fingertips: where you are able to shape and shift your life through the internal intelligence that is uniquely yours.

Mind Makeover

Today in your journaling, think about your unique strengths. Take just 5 or 10 minutes to do this—don't overthink it. Attempt to see yourself as an outsider would.

1. (In your personality) Ask yourself: Am I funny? Am I charismatic? Am I thoughtful? Am I compassionate? Write down anything that comes to mind.

2. (In your work) Ask yourself: What are my unique strengths in my work? Am I hardworking? Am I creative? Am I good at working with other people?

3. (In your personal connections) Ask your-

self: What are my unique strengths in my capacity for love or connection within my community? My family?

....

TODAY'S MANTRA:
I am brilliant.

....

Building Awareness

Do you find today's mantra a bit hard to accept? Today, notice how your intelligence emerges through your unique strengths, both in your work and in your life. Notice those moments of interaction or completion as a sense of genius. Think, *This is my strength. This is my intelligence, and my unique ability to contribute through that intelligence.* Notice your unique intelligence as it comes out both in how you handle your cravings for foods but also how you do your job—are you using your intelligence to its highest potential? Notice how you connect with your friends, colleagues, family, with strong relationships being a crystal-clear reflection of your unique contributions.

DAY 12: LOVE

....

"I deserve love."

Today we focus on our belief in our own innate goodness.

We all make mistakes. Sometimes we wish we could go back and do things differently. Even though we're all human, we have a tendency to judge ourselves harshly, as if we could be perfect machines. This judgment has the power to really change our perspective of ourselves.

We face choices every day—and those choices and our reactions to them sculpt our lives in many ways. How we choose to respond to our own personal triggers changes everything. When we act in ways that don't support our highest ideals, we can feel guilt and start to put too much pressure on ourselves. But it's necessary to forgive ourselves when we don't live up to our own expectations. The most important thing about this forgiveness is the healing that we do in just acknowledging the mistake.

The reality is, we couldn't go through life and not make mistakes. Mistakes really are valuable, allowing us to grow and learn from our experiences. When we make them, that is human nature—whether we fall off a diet, fall short of our workout or career goals, or disappoint a loved one. How do we love ourselves regardless? Sometimes it becomes difficult to believe that we deserve love.

We all have flaws, blind spots; we make errors and hold regret. Obviously, we would like to avoid these perceived failures, but our ability to look at those mistakes and learn from them rather than judge ourselves and put ourselves down is what's important. It's also possible to consider how our choices relate to the valuing of our own intelligence. Our ideas about who we are define and change us. For many of us, myself included, it often takes many failures—whether in relationships or jobs—to figure out what we really need. What do we really want? What makes us tick?

After a certain number of failed attempts to lose pounds, only to gain them back, it becomes harder and harder to look yourself in the eye, to believe what is true—that we all deserve to be loved. We then tend to close ourselves off due to our insecurities and failures. We find it difficult to share ourselves with others, and that carries over into how we react to others and how we interact with ourselves.

I think we get stuck on the idea that when big things go wrong, they are defining moments. But defining moments happen at any time; they are constantly happening. We have the ability to reflect on any moment and decide how we want to define ourselves. Although there may be failures, we have the potential to have a defining moment at any point in our lives.

We all deserve love. We all mess up. The two aren't mutually exclusive. Messing up doesn't mean we don't deserve love. The ability to face our mistakes and still believe we deserve love is the foundation for wellness and longevity. On any wellness plan, we're going to stumble at points. But we must remind ourselves that that is human nature, rather than a shortcoming. Let's acknowledge that even after failure or regret or going off the wagon, we still deserve love.

7-MINUTE MEDITATION

7

Coming back to your observer stance, settle in comfortably. As you begin, notice your breathing and begin to attend to the experience inside your body today. Start to consider the sensation behind your experience of love. What does it feel like in your body—is it warm or cold, heavy or light, expanding or contracting? Notice which parts of your body feel more connected to this feeling.

As you inhale, breathing naturally, visualize love coming into your body. Then, on the exhale, visualize allowing that love to settle into your bones.

Imagine all the cells of your body receiving love. If you have trouble connecting to some areas, spend a little extra time on those and bring your awareness to that area to see if you can feed it even more. Just take the love in and allow your cells to bathe in it. Inhale and breathe love into your cells; exhale and let it settle deep into your bones. Continue this throughout today's meditation.

Mind Makeover

Today we're going to dive deep and get real about any sense of failure you may be holding on to in your life.

1. What are your biggest regrets or failures?
2. How have they defined you—or how have you allowed them to define you?
3. Is it possible to change your perspective

and see them as learning opportunities and a platform for growth, inspiration, or transformation? (I know this is a very hard one. Just to be able to sit with the list you created and look at those experiences is difficult work. We may talk offhandedly about our mistakes, but we rarely look at them this deeply. Mere complaints about our missteps can remain somewhat shallow—but truly facing the reality of their consequences is a little bit harder.)

....

TODAY'S MANTRA:
I deserve love.

....

Building Awareness

Really spend some time with this mantra today. Notice when the mantra is easier to accept and feels lighter, and also notice any resistance, and in which settings you feel that resistance. Notice how the belief that you deserve love—or the lack of belief in it—affects your interactions with others: Does it help you feel more patient, more tolerant? More worried or scared? Does it give you confidence? Drag you down? Also, notice how this mantra impacts your relationship with food, and in what ways. Dig deep.

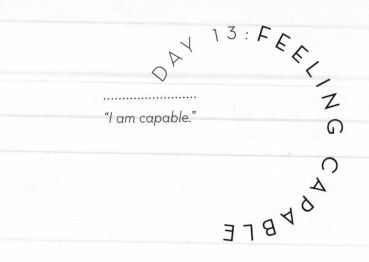

DAY 13: FEELING CAPABLE

....
"I am capable."

Today is about committing to this program and seeing it through.

Sometimes being healthy can seem like an impossible task. We hear about so many different ideas and programs and theories on weight loss and health and wellness. I think we all can come to a place where we learn so much, and so much that is contradictory, that the quest of becoming "completely healthy" seems futile.

For me, this came up when I graduated from Chinese medicine school. Like so many others who've graduated from naturopathic or other holistic health programs, I went through a phase of recovery afterward. After four or five years of learning about all of the things that are bad or good for you in this world, you just feel a bit paralyzed. You can put so much pressure on yourself to do every single specific thing you learned about that the result can almost be worse for your health.

After this period of paralysis, I started giving myself permission to not be 100 percent healthy. We get stuck in this idea that to be really healthy, we have to be perfect. *I can't ever eat something bad. I can't ever do something bad.* Everything we learn about self-care here can turn into judgment, which can make the whole sense of despair and paralysis even worse.

Remember when we talked about stress not necessarily being bad for you—it's your belief about the stress that matters? That same logic follows here: It's our attachment to the thought that certain things are bad that gives them their power over us. We need to develop our ability to be okay with not being 100 percent perfect. In my experience, this is the hardest part of leading a healthy life: fully embracing moderation.

In yoga, Buddhism, and other spiritual traditions, we hear about the path of moderation. We humans find it so easy to go to extremes, we'll do a grapefruit juice diet or a fast—that all-or-nothing approach feels good because we don't have to doubt or explore any gray areas. The instructions are clear, and they help us feel secure.

The hard part is not the actual following of the extreme diets but recognizing that they do not reflect reality—acknowledging that, at some point, we need to come back to moderation and resume the flexibility necessary to live in the real world. And hopefully we come to a place of understanding that it is that flexibility—and not a stubborn, unyielding adherence to dogma—that makes us strong.

So how do we avoid being completely overwhelmed by all we know about what's good for us and what's not good for us? How do we choose where to start a "healthy" life? How do we know when enough is enough?

One place to start is with the science. Research has found that committing to small changes over long periods can be much better for our health than big changes that are short-lived. Big ups and downs in weight cause stress in the body and may actually be more detrimental to our health than remaining at a steady weight. Just understanding the danger in extremes can help us recognize that absolute perfection is not required to be healthy—in fact, it's not even necessarily healthy (or possible).

One of the most important aspects of health is your social life. A glass of wine or a lovely dinner with friends can be part of that social connection, which can have greater impact on our long-term health than a juice fast. Dr. Dean Ornish, a legendary cardiologist and nutrition researcher, amassed a large body of research on the health benefits of a low-fat, vegetarian diet and how it decreased heart disease. Interestingly, his follow-up work looked closely at social connection and family support, and he found that these social resources had an even greater impact on heart health than diet.

Mindfulness is the best way to tease out the benefits in this balance between social connection and what we eat. We can think about and ask ourselves, *How many days a week is it okay to go out to drink wine for the social connection? How much am I in need of a healthy diet?*

If we learn to pay attention and listen to what the body needs, we can have a much healthier, happier, and less stressful relationship with our diet and what we do to remain healthy. *Do I need to just stay at home and be quiet, since I've been going out a lot? Do I need to eat some clean, simple, healthy foods, or have I been too strict with myself in my diet and my exercise? Maybe today is a good day to go out and have a glass of wine, but not five.*

When we plant those seeds, we are able to make some simple, attainable changes that we commit to and follow through on. We recognize that these changes don't necessarily have to be what we do our entire lives. They don't need to seem "life-changing." In actuality, true life change is the accumulation of the small things to which we can commit over time. In the same way, we can give ourselves permission to simply *enjoy* from time to time, while realizing that those moments are healthy as well. Committing to simple changes and not having to be perfect make us healthier all around. And help us feel capable.

7-MINUTE MEDITATION

7

Today's meditation is about steadiness. I think the hard part of moderation, or committing to simple changes and not having to be perfect, is feeling steady in that commitment. This meditation is a simple way of keying in to the steadiness already within you.

Start in a sitting position. When you close your eyes, just notice the heaviness of your legs and pelvis as that steadying component. Think about the steadiness of the base of our sitting position, the legs and pelvis and hips, and the stability that creates. Now shift your attention to the natural changes in the breath, the resemblance to the fluctuations in our lives, the ups and downs. Notice the ability of these two experiences, the ups and downs of our breath, to coexist and support each other.

Mind Makeover

Today I want you to pick three small changes that you will commit to for the remainder of this retreat—meditation and two others. (If they suit you, I hope you will choose to continue them after as well, but this commitment is just for the next 8 days.)

Key word here: *small*. Keeping these small will help you follow through on your commitment to yourself. In your journal, write them out in this format: "I will _____."

Here are some suggestions:

- Drink two extra glasses of water a day.
- Do yoga for 30 minutes at least once this week.
- Get up from my desk every hour.
- Walk for 20 minutes three times this week.

Make them very simple and attainable but specific. You're working to strengthen your commitment muscle to attain your goals.

....

TODAY'S MANTRA:

I am capable.

....

Building Awareness

Today I would like you to train your attention on accomplishing all three of your goals. You've already done the first—your meditation. The remaining two will be your focus for the day ahead.

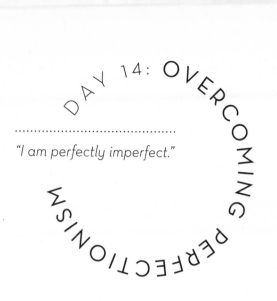

"I am perfectly imperfect."

As humans, we find it so much easier to see our flaws than our strengths. The reality is, we all have imperfections. Even airbrushed models and celebrities have a long list of flaws, both visible and then, magically, not. But our flaws are what make us humans. Without them we'd be just robots. We'd all look the same. We'd all have perfect noses and perfect skin and perfect butts, and we'd all walk around perfectly happy. Life would be incredibly boring. Even if we were to get the perfect body and perfect hair and perfect personality, there would always be problems underneath this surface perfection.

Our imperfections are our humanity—they are how we connect to one another. We've all experienced this during a time of struggle. We let our guard down and are able to connect more deeply with the people around us and have those relationship-defining moments with friends or significant others. Those imperfections create the opening for us to connect, for us to recognize one another's humanity. They are what earn us the meaning and the depth in our lives.

Knowing this, is it possible to see your flaws as the imperfections that make you perfectly imperfect? And as part of what allows you to connect more deeply to the world around you? Whether that's freckles or cellulite or love handles—or just your quirky personality? That goofy laugh, or the gap between your teeth?

As much as I want to fix or cover up my supposed flaws, I'm happy knowing that my weak points can be my strengths. The more light I can shed on my flaw or imperfection, the less it can torture me. I will never be perfect. What I can do is recognize how these qualities affect me now, and choose to consciously create new patterns to live by with a commitment to simply be aware of the darkness. At that point I can clearly see what is real.

I'm sure you've heard the old adage that we cannot love anyone else until we love ourselves. But I think it's a myth that we should love ourselves, at least in the way this implies. Sometimes the concept of self-love can feel so artificial as to be impossible, especially right after a difficult loss or failure. If we dig a little, we can uncover feelings of worthlessness that can make even rudimentary self-love seem out of our reach. I remember struggling so much as a kid, being teased really badly by my peers and always wanting to please my parents. When I got older, in moments when I felt like a failure, I started to realize that this was the same dark place I'd experienced when I was younger. All the internal bodily sensations and responses felt the same. When I realized that my suffering had always been a reflection of something pulling the trigger on my sense of worthlessness, I was able to recognize how this same feeling was showing up in my present life.

Maybe it's not as much about self-love as we think. Maybe it's about just sitting with unease and finding that we don't die from discomfort. Perhaps it's simply about acknowledging and sitting in the unease long enough for it to loosen its grip on us. About acknowledging that we have flaws and become okay with that thought. Healthy self-love is more about seeing ourselves as we are, "flaws" and all, and recognizing that these qualities make us human and that they allow us to connect more deeply with the people around us. This commitment to living with your eyes open allows you to recognize your patterns and choose a life that feeds you, rather than grasping for a cliché of self-love to patch the problem. Living this way removes the illusion that someday all your problems will disappear. In its place is the awareness that you have the power to slowly carve new patterns to replace your habitual ones. Knowing that this flaw or issue may continue to rear its head and torment you, again and again, you can have the awareness to notice how it affects you, and you can choose to rewrite the story.

7-MINUTE MEDITATION

7

Today, I want you to visualize your imperfections. I want you to pick one in particular that really stands out to you, whether it's physical or an aspect of your personality. It might be your nose or your belly, or maybe your impatience or lack of assertion. For example, if you feel that you're too impatient, or you get angry too quickly—what's really at work there? Are you uncomfortable with feeling anger? If it's your nose or your belly, can you imagine what you might be like if every part of our bodies were the same, "perfect" shape? What if these imperfections are just reflections of you? As you meditate, see if it's possible to acknowledge that imperfection as a sign of your humanness, as a sign of your being alive. Notice what it feels like to be alive in your body with your particular nose or your particular impatience, or whatever your quality is. Notice your ability to sit down for your meditation and notice your breath, regardless of your body or your imperfections. Notice this connection to being an observer, how it relates to the experience of life and what it feels like to be alive. And notice this one imperfection as a symbol of your humanness, and your gratitude for your life.

Mind Makeover

For today's journaling:

1. Write down what you consider to be your physical imperfections. Pick three that stand out. How would your life be different without them, and what would it look like?

2. Without them, would you still be you? Whether your imperfections are freckles

or cellulite or the shape of your nose, or the stretch marks from your baby, consider how they have played a role in crafting you. Many women learn this lesson from motherhood, as they change before and after the birth of their children. They become these nurturing, motherly, beautiful women. Would you want to give that up? Just to lose your love handles? Would it still be you? Would it still be your life? Would all of the things that you know as your life still be part of that?

....

TODAY'S MANTRA:
I am perfectly imperfect.

....

Building Awareness

Consider: Can you change your perspective—just for today? Just for today, notice your imperfections as perfectly you, as an aspect of your humanness. Some of us have trouble resisting the siren call of our own negativity, but can you make the commitment to yourself, just for one day, to love your imperfections as an aspect of who you are, an aspect that is worthy of love? Some find it hard to imagine not hating their stomachs or their love handles. But what if you gave yourself permission to just let it go for one day—what does that feel like? Explore that during the day ahead.

....

"I am vibrant."

One of the hardest things for many of my patients is to get to a point in their healing journey where they can experience what it's like to feel good. Most of us go through life with an array of pain and discomfort and disconnection from our own health. And it becomes so hard just to remember what it feels like to feel good, to feel well, to feel comfortable in your own skin. But to lose weight and get healthy, we first have to believe in our own capacity to heal. Our capacity to get better. What if our belief in our ability to heal and lose weight was the precursor to our weight loss? Just the belief itself?

Our perspective, the places we choose to place our attention and our attitude toward that attention, can have a big impact on our physical health. One study published in the *Journal of Personality and Social Psychology* found that those participants who were asked to count their blessings in their journal once a week for 9 weeks had much better health outcomes than those who were asked to document their burdens or simply record events in their lives. Overall, those who counted their blessings felt better about their lives as a whole and were more optimistic regarding their expectations for the upcoming week. They reported fewer physical complaints and spending significantly more time exercising. When the researchers bumped it up to once a day for weeks, they found that daily counting of blessings also helped people to feel significantly more grateful, more likely to have helped someone else, and to enjoy better moods (using words such as *attentive, determined, energetic, enthusiastic, excited, interested, joyful,* and *strong*).[1] Then researchers tested a similar intervention with people who endured chronic pain, and they found that simply counting blessings increased their total hours of sleep, helped them feel better and more refreshed upon waking, decreased their physical pain, and increased their functional status.

Can you imagine a life without debilitating pain,

physical or emotional? Can you imagine a life without weight as a limiting factor? Where you can be free to be happy and healthy? Think about how much of our lives we experience pain and discomfort and how much our health is burdened by these experiences. Although it may be difficult, or a distant memory, really focus on remembering what it's like to feel well. *Especially* if it's been a long time. You have that knowledge within you. Remember, our belief in our capacity to heal is the root of all progress.

Today's meditation will be very simple— but the challenge is to make it as vivid and real as possible. Today you will be visualizing yourself in vibrant health.

Begin by noticing the sense of vibrant health inside of your body in this moment. Notice what it feels like to be vibrantly alive. What does the sensation feel like in your body? What does the shape of your body feel like? What is the quality of your body? Is there a particular place in your body that feels this vibrant health? Focus your thoughts there and imagine this sense of vibrant health flooding into the rest of you.

Then I want you to picture yourself with this sense of vibrant health as you go through the rest of your day. Picture it vividly and notice how you carry yourself differently. Notice how you interact with people differently. Most of all, notice how you feel differently, during and at the end of your day, with this sense of vibrant health. Do you manage your energy in new ways? End your meditation by bringing your awareness back to what it feels like to embrace the experience of vibrant health in this moment.

Mind Makeover

Before you begin your journal exercises, I want you to think of three positive things—either about your life's path, your relationships, your job, the world, anything. You will think of those things throughout the day today.

Now, much like the participants in the study I described previously, we are going to let the good settle into our bones with this writing exercise.

1. Think of three positive things you will experience during the day to come. What are you looking forward to?

2. What would it feel like to be vibrantly healthy in your day today? What aspects of your life would be different? Write down, in detail, how you feel now and what it would feel like to be healthy— what would have to change in order for you to feel that way? Look at the obvious things, but dig for a few subtle things, too. How do you feel in your skin? How does your body affect how you're acting? How do you connect with the people around you?

....

TODAY'S MANTRA:
I am vibrant.

....

Building Awareness

Today I'd like you to tap in to or visualize this awareness of vibrant health at least three times during the course of the day, for just a few moments. Maybe even set reminders on your phone, and when those times come, close your eyes and remind yourself to tap in to that feeling of vitality. Ask yourself, *What does it feel like to be healthy in this moment? What does it feel like to be alive?*

Then, before you go to bed this evening, I want you to recall the three positive things you came up with earlier today. Repeat this process every day and night for the remaining 6 days of the program.

DAY 16: EMBRACING YOUR BEAUTY

"I am awesome as I am."

Sometimes when we're at this stage in a new program, it can be easy to feel stuck. Once we begin to make some progress, we want to look like the pretty pictures we see. When reality falls short of that unrealistic expectation, instead of seeing ourselves clearly or acknowledging how far we have come, we just see what's wrong. But your natural beauty is with you always and does not depend on what's on the scale.

It's easy to compare ourselves with pictures and constantly want to be better. It's possible to use these images in a healthy way, inspiring us to positive change. But it's a fine line between looking to images of other people for inspiration and seeing them as a mandate to change ourselves. At what stage do we begin to feel the need to change certain things about ourselves in order to feel beautiful?

Many women have a morning beauty routine—applying makeup, fixing hair, choosing clothes. But this routine can morph into mandatory prep, what we *have* to go through in order to be presentable to the world. We don't even consider leaving the house without it.

I went through a phase of loving fake eyelashes. A friend talked me into trying them, and I started going to a salon to have them applied professionally, and they'd stay on for a month.

When I first got them, I was totally infatuated. I loved how they looked and how easy they were. I'd wake up and look like I had makeup on! But at some point, the lashes would start falling off. And when they did, I felt like something was missing. I became dependent on going every few weeks to get them touched up.

After a few cycles of this, I got to a point of dependence, feeling as though I *needed* the eyelashes to be pretty. And every time they'd start to fall off, I'd start to think to myself, *Oh, my eyes look so boring.* Makeup can be very similar—we get used to looking at ourselves in a certain way, and we get to a place where we *need* to "put the face on." Or, if you don't wear makeup, maybe it's about your clothes. Or the way you do your hair. We have certain rituals we develop as mandatory precursors to being ready to face the world.

Yet we all have a natural beauty that shines outwardly but starts from inside of us. It might be our smile, or the glow of our skin, or our white teeth, strong legs, clear eyes. We all have some aspect of our physical body that radiates natural beauty in some unique way. Accentuating and calling attention to our beauty is a tricky line to walk. When is enough enough?

I'm not suggesting that the answer is to stop adorning our physical body forever. However, that firm belief that we must never go to work without makeup—are we certain of that? Who made that decision, and do we have to abide by it? We have many expectations of how we need to look for certain roles in our lives. How do we know they're valid?

I can't say I'll never put fake eyelashes on again. Nor do I need to become a hippie and stop shaving and give up makeup or wear only organic clothes. I love my clothes and my jewelry. I love fashion. To me fashion is also an art. But when it becomes a necessity so that we feel presentable, it can leave us feeling a bit empty.

Today, take a closer look at your beautification habits and consider whether your routine has become a mandatory ritual, something that you *must* do to feel presentable to the world. Consider such rituals as another way you bury yourself, another way to potentially cover up your natural beauty. Can you notice the role that you play in disconnecting from your natural beauty? Is it possible to see yourself and your natural beauty clearly, to see how far you've already come, not just in how you look but in your shifting perspective?

As you settle into meditation, take stock for a bit. During your meditation, notice the changes in your ability to sit and observe what you've experienced thus far. Become aware of your perception of the experience in your body.

Then, consider your perception of yourself in the world as you just sit and observe again. How do you see yourself? How do you carry yourself? What message does this tell you about your belief in your beauty?

Start to hone in on your natural beauty—think about the aspects of your physical body that you feel most proud of. It could be the shininess of your hair, the softness of your skin, the sparkle in your eyes—even the shape of your feet. Notice what it feels like to appreciate your natural assets. Then visualize how you might carry yourself differently with that appreciation, when you consider it your unique natural beauty. Consider how you might move through your day differently with this awareness.

Then come back to your breath and notice if the experience in your body has changed. Continue to notice this awareness in your body as you observe your breath. When the timer goes off, turn immediately to your journal.

Mind Makeover

Reflect on these questions in your journal:

1. Write down your natural beauty assets. What do *you* see as your natural points of beauty? Is it your nose or smile or legs or eyes or hair—or something specific like the length of your legs or the strength of your legs, your posture or the color of your hair?

2. How do you hide or appreciate those things? Is there a way to accentuate them naturally?

....

TODAY'S MANTRA:

I am awesome as I am.

....

Building Awareness

Today your challenge is to think of one or two ways in which you can naturally accentuate your beauty points, such as drink more water, brush your hair until it shines, or take a relaxing bath with essential oils, ways that are totally different from your normal routine. I'd also like you to look at any of your regular routines that suggest you must *put on* certain things—clothes, jewelry, makeup—to look pretty.

I think every woman can relate to the idea of adding things in order to enhance beauty, rather than taking things away to reveal the natural beauty that's already there. For example, maybe one of your routines has been to put on eye cream at night. You may have a tendency to tell yourself, *I have to put on this eye cream, otherwise my eyes are going to start to look ugly,* or *I like my eyes, but if I don't use my eye cream every night and wear makeup every day, people will see me differently.*

How many things do we pour on our skin based on advertisements that basically say, "If you put this on, you will have radiant skin; if you don't, you will look old." While buying lotions and makeup, many have also bought in to the thought *I'm going to put this on to be beautiful*—but what does it tell us about ourselves, if we subconsciously buy in to these messages? And what does that leave us feeling at the end of the day when we strip it all away?

Think of my fake eyelashes: At a certain point, I became dependent on them to feel "beautiful." The eyelashes *are* beautiful and fun, and that was fine until I realized I needed them to feel beautiful and started to examine what that was telling me about what was underneath the eyelashes. What are the things that we do on a regular basis that program us to feel we need something more—high heels, designer scents, dyed hair, facial contouring, spray tan—to be beautiful?

Today, see what you can let go of in your routine. This bit of "less" doesn't need to be extreme— you don't have to go to work without any makeup or not doing your hair. Simply notice it as a way of shifting your perspective so you recognize that the way you present yourself in the world also sends subconscious messages about your belief in your innate beauty. Maybe your beauty is in your skin or your smile—not the layer of makeup you add every day. Maybe you don't need to straighten your hair, or pencil in your eyebrows, or wear those high heels today. Maybe you could just wear simpler clothes today and, instead, appreciate the beauty in your smile.

What are the ways you can accentuate your natural beauty today?

....

"I am sexy."

Yesterday we talked about seeing and celebrating our natural beauty. Today we'll talk about our sexy side, something each one of us has, no matter our age or partner status.

Sexiness carries over to many aspects of our lives. Being able to tap in to our sex appeal is not only great for self-confidence, it also greatly enhances our relationships with partners and even our physical health. Chemicals released during sex—such as endorphins and oxytocin—not only help us feel fantastic and euphoric, they can also help us avoid certain chronic diseases and even live longer.

We all go through a time when it's really difficult to see ourselves as sexy. Obviously our level of sex drive can change throughout the month, based on hormonal fluctuations. But I'm talking about a bigger issue here. We get so used to living with ourselves, it can be hard to remember all of our alluring, attractive aspects sometimes. Guys might not struggle with this as much as women—women can get disconnected from our bodies and forget how to embrace our sexiness. Some of us find it much easier than others to see ourselves as sexy.

Let today be a reminder that sexy is not an aspect of how we look. Sexiness shines through our eyes and how we carry ourselves, and certainly how we treat other people. There's a big difference between feeling sexy and being flirtatious, which is where many of us get confused. Sexy is a sense of powerful pleasure and desire that we exude from within; flirtatious is about soliciting feedback from another person.

Have you ever had the experience of meeting someone really beautiful but then gotten to know her—and found out she is not nice? All of a sudden you see that person entirely differently—she starts to look kind of ugly to you.

Then you might meet a person who seems kind of average—but his personality and the way he connects and fits with you is so appealing, and as you get to know him, you see this incredibly sexy side of him. His face, his whole being then becomes irresistibly cute.

Sexiness is in our confidence and in our step; it's in the way we linger and laugh. The glow in our skin. The radiance in our smile. Sex appeal is really just the way that we move and connect with people and ourselves.

For most of my life I saw myself as kind of a nerd. I'd be off in a corner somewhere with my nose in a book and hardly thought of myself as sexy. I certainly never saw myself as a role model for sexy. But then I started working with clothing designer Kira Karmazin on her very beautiful, glamorous line of yoga clothes, KiraGrace. Kira had been a longtime yoga student of mine when she started the business. I loved her yoga clothes, so when she approached me, of course I wanted to help.

The first time I showed up for a photo shoot, I felt so awkward and uncomfortable. I had no idea *what* I was doing—I wasn't a model! But I didn't want to let her down, so I did the best I could.

Somehow, after several of these shoots and a lot of encouragement from her team, I felt more natural and easy. I started to have fun with it. And now, when I look back over the past few years, I can see how much the pictures have changed since that first shoot, and it fascinates me. It's not my physical appearance that's so different. But doing these sexy shoots with her made me step out of my comfort zone. I used to look at the pictures and pick myself apart—I've always hated my big cheeks. But as I started to embrace the sexiness that came through when I began to believe in my own inner beauty, the pictures changed immensely. How much of what we see as sexy in the media is really just a reflection of the model's confidence? I can clearly see that as I've become more comfortable and confident with the modeling, I've grown to embody my personal beauty in a way that shines through as sexy, even with all my nerdy habits.

Sexiness is a belief in ourselves, a confidence that comes as we learn to trust our natural beauty and allure. But there are many ways that we almost shame ourselves to shut down our sexiness. Especially if you're a professional woman or a mother, being a little sexy is maybe okay—but there's a subtle societal demand that we keep it under restraint, especially once we have a partner or get married. Yet I think sexiness is such an important part of our emotional and physical health—we need to allow ourselves to step into it and embody it, without feeling shame or other limitations.

When I look at those yoga modeling photos now, I can see the difference between my first and my more recent photos more clearly than the average person can. But I'm so grateful to those photos for showing me how the difference in my comfort level could be seen and witnessed by those around me. They made the intangible tangible. And now I'm eager to help you fully own your own beauty and sexiness.

Begin with observing your breath, observing your experience of your breathing. Then, after you settle in, consider and visualize what it feels like to be sexy. Really embody it. What is the sensation? What does it feel like to visualize yourself as sexy? Is it difficult to even visualize? How does it feel to live in your body with this awareness?

Notice this experience of being sexy as an extension of your natural beauty that we looked at yesterday, but now with a sense of confidence behind it. Notice how your belief in your own natural beauty, as well as your innate intelligence, merge together to create this bone-deep sexy quality. How might your relationship with your body change with this awareness? How might your relationships change with this sense of confidence that you exude?

As you continue to notice your breathing, sit there and notice what it feels like to be sexy. Notice the shape and the texture and the sensations in your body as you contemplate the importance of this mental state.

Mind Makeover

In today's journaling, we'll dig a little further into the idea of sexiness:

1. How can you embrace sexy—whether it's in your looks, your clothes, the way you talk, or the way you connect with people? Your smile? Your glow? How can you embrace that essential sexy feeling? How can you acknowledge your inherent sexiness, without having to flirt, and just be aware and confident and embrace it?

2. Look back at your answers and consider: Are they dependent on other people? How can you separate your sense of sexiness from having people notice you? How can you completely disconnect it from what the world around you sees or thinks? Just notice what it feels like to be sexy from your own perspective.

....

TODAY'S MANTRA:

I am sexy.

....

Building Awareness

Today, visualize yourself as sexy. For some of us, it may sound like an easy assignment. But for those of us who have a tendency to see our flaws but not our strengths, this will be challenging—we often miss how sexy we are naturally. Wear something that reminds you of this, not by putting on a ton of makeup but how you inhabit your body, how you speak and carry yourself with confidence. Maybe even lighten up on the makeup (or leave it behind completely) and see if you can radiate beauty from the inside out, through your smile, your conversation, your glow, and your appreciation for life. How do you carry yourself differently when you feel sexy? Can you embrace what that feels like today without having to cover anything up?

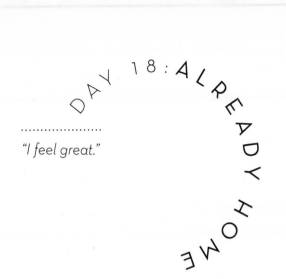

DAY 18: ALREADY HOME

....

"I feel great."

Remember Leslie in chapter 1? She was so disciplined and dedicated. She'd done everything she could to lose weight, but nothing worked—until she started to meditate and see herself as a lighter person. That opened up a channel in her body and mind to make that image her reality.

One of the tricky things about losing weight is that our brains must be able to visualize us at a healthy weight before our bodies can make it so. Once we've been overweight for a while, it becomes really difficult to see ourselves at a healthy weight, or even contemplate what it would feel like. We forget what it's like to feel comfortable in our body, to be able to move easily and comfortably through our lives. But once we're able to visualize that, our nervous system can get to work to try to create it—just like the dictum "Believe it, be it."

Studies have shown that once we visualize a goal, and we *believe* we will achieve it, we start to consciously and subconsciously change our behavior to create that reality. A recent analysis of sixty-six studies that looked at how we imagine our goals and the plans we make to reach them found that this "theory of planned behavior" can have a major positive impact in many struggles we encounter, with reductions in socially undesirable behavior, binge drinking, risky driving, and sugar consumption.[2] Another study found that simply planning to eat more fruits and vegetables did, indeed, cause first-year college students to eat over 40 percent more than they did at the start of the study.[3]

Today's focus is very simple. If your aim is to lose weight, today you will create a visual image of yourself already at your healthy body weight. I believe this is the crux of long-term change: To bring that goal to fruition, your brain has to be able to wrap itself around a believable image of you achieving this goal. I want you to develop the ability to notice your potential to be healthy, to achieve a normal weight, and to embody the concept of coming home to yourself.

Today's meditation is about seeing yourself at a healthy weight and it's probably one of the most pivotal meditations I've used with my patients over the years.

After you settle into a comfortable seat, come back to your breathing. Begin by noticing the sensations of the outline of your body, your belly, your hips, your legs. Then turn your mind toward creating this image of yourself at a healthy weight.

Specifically, what does it feel like? See if you can picture yourself in your mind's eye at this weight. (It might be difficult to imagine, but do your best.) What does it look like? Notice the sensations in this healthy body, visualize how you would move in your body. Would you walk differently or carry yourself differently? Even something simple like getting in and out of your car, how would that feel? Would it feel different when you get out of bed? Would your clothes fit differently? Notice how you might move through your day differently. How do you talk differently? Do you interact differently? How does your body feel throughout your day?

Picture yourself going through a full day—whether you're reading this at night and thinking about tomorrow, or you're reading this in the morning and thinking about the day ahead. Really envision all the detail, but notice everything that feels different. How do you sit at your desk? How do you walk? Stand? Try to be as vivid as possible. Then come back to noticing your breath and holding all of those qualities in your body now. Keep those pictures in your mind's eye as you continue through your day.

Mind Makeover

Today's journaling will help us crystallize this image and hold on to it, so we can bring it into reality.

1. Once you've really settled on your image, consider: What does it feel like to live in this healthy image of your body? Not just visually but practically, too—what does it mean to move through your day in this body?

2. Write down all the positive changes you will feel—in your body, mind, stress level, physical health, relationships, work success—everything.

TODAY'S MANTRA:
I feel great.

Building Awareness

As you go through your day, come back to this image at least three times. Hold it in your brain for just a few moments, close your eyes, and bring your awareness back to what it feels like to inhabit this healthy image of your body. You are literally shifting the nervous system and creating that touch point. When your brain visualizes a trait or quality, your nervous system can go to work trying to bring it to fruition. If you are unable to even visualize these changes, your weight loss or life goals will be nearly impossible to achieve. You've got to believe it to achieve it. Spend today visualizing these changes as vividly as possible.

....

"My inner glow makes me radiant."

Today we are wrapping up a progression that we've made through the last few days. First we looked at our "flaws," then at our potential for health. Then we looked at our potential for natural beauty and for being sexy. Yesterday we looked at our potential to inhabit and grow into a healthy image of our body. Today we'll look at our inner glow and the potential that radiates from our internal strength—our character.

Character is the source of our inner strengths, and it exudes from within to create a sense of radiance. Whether that character is based in our work or our ethics or our family life, our spiritual life or our creative life, that cohesion of intention and action

creates integrity. That inner glow comes from this integrity, this commitment to what is really meaningful to us.

Integrity is a word that gets thrown around a lot.
The dictionary defines *integrity* as the state of being
whole and undivided. To me, integrity is the ability to
have cohesion in what we do and align our acts with
our purpose and strengths. It is the ability to do what
we say and to lead by example. It is a personal commitment to what is meaningful to us: to be clear in
our purpose and keep our priorities in line with that.

In this modern, disjointed, unfocused world, how
can we redouble our efforts to maintain our integrity?

Today I want you to think about your own integrity. Look at the list of personal strengths we gathered
on day 11 and notice how these strengths contribute
to your inner radiance. At this stage in your program, what are your given strengths of personality
and character, both at work and in your personal life?
And what effect do they have on your perception of
your life? How can you utilize these strengths to access this very deepest layer, the reflection of your
inner glow?

Throughout my life, it has been really important

to me to stay true to what I find meaningful. Whether it's work or family, so many responsibilities pull us in so many directions, asking us to be so many different things at once. To me, integrity is being able to commit to what's important to us, and realign the rest of our own world around those ideals.

Our ability to commit to what we believe in, whether the road is rocky or easy, is integrity. There's not a judgment of one road being right or wrong—that integrity is unique to you. And today I want to talk about being able to hold true to that in order to find the inner radiance that comes from clarity of purpose as well as the strengths that we began looking at on day 11.

The meditation for day 19 is really simple, but it's also really powerful. Sometimes the simplest meditation can be the most challenging. Begin by coming back to the observer's mind-set, just as you have before. Notice the sensations in your body. Notice the natural pace of your breath and the life inherent in your breath. Now, visualize your inner beauty as a quality that lies just under your skin. Imagine that sense of inner beauty coming from underneath the skin right as it manifests on the outer skin and shines off the exterior of the body. Notice this inner glow as it comes from beneath the skin to create a sense of radiance on the surface of the body from the inside. Continue your meditation with your awareness on this quality of inner beauty as you allow yourself to sit in stillness and watch the breath moving naturally and enhancing this inner glow.

Mind Makeover

Today let's revisit our strengths:

1. What are your inner strengths, both in work and in life? What are your skills, specifically how they intersect with your personality and character? What effect do these qualities have on your perception of your life? How can you utilize these strengths in your work or in other areas of your life?

2. Review your strengths list from day 11. Add to it, if needed. How do these strengths contribute to your radiance, in your appearance and your interactions?

....

TODAY'S MANTRA:

My inner glow makes me radiant.

....

Building Awareness

We've been talking about inner beauty, radiance, sexiness—and now we're pulling it together with your unique contributions and your integrity.

Throughout your day, notice how your inner strengths contribute to your outer radiance. Notice how you interact, how you talk, the confidence you exude, or your sense of integrity and the way that transmits your inner radiance out into the world. Notice how that focus on integrity strengthens your presence, your confidence, and your ability to connect with people.

Consider how your external beauty also comes from your personal strengths. Many find it comforting to realize that outer beauty is not all that dependent on weight or makeup or visible assets, that so much comes through a person's character and integrity.

Consider this in both your work and your family life. How do I lead by example? When you have children, you're constantly being watched—how do you lead them by example at any given moment of the day with integrity? How do your integrity and radiance contribute to your ability to see your goals through and continue taking steps toward your healthy body weight?

Notice how your inner strengths contribute to your outer radiance today.

DAY 20: COMMITMENT

....

"I am committed to feeling great."

Our health is constantly changing. There are never two moments when the cells in our body are exactly the same. This mind-bending reality has pros and cons.

Pros: We can change.

Cons: Those changes could be downhill.

Obviously, our health requires maintenance and will always take some fine-tuning. But the pro is that we can, at any moment, steer that change in the direction we want.

Day 20 is about committing to your health as an important foundation of the endurance of this work. Commitment is the ability to not just see this program through for the 21 days but developing the ability to see it through the long term, so you can maintain health. Your health is not a static state—it is a process that happens over the course of the years, rather than the days or the weeks, of our lives. In this way, our health is just the collection of small habits that we make a decision to commit to long-term.

In our lives, change is constant. We are always riding a wave between our current lives and our potential lives—our surfboard is our ability to steer that change. Mindfulness is a tool to help us steer more steadily and consistently. Mindfulness helps us pay attention and notice when things are starting to veer off course. Mindfulness helps us use our awareness to shift our perspective, to notice our relationship with food or with exercise or with our bodies. To maintain a health program, the only thing required is a commitment to that mindful awareness and to notice that you can steer your mindful awareness in a different direction at any moment. Whether you're increasing your awareness of your physical health, food, and exercise, your mental health, spiritual health, or your outlook and perspective, there is no end point—there is only a process of continuing to look. Even if you've followed this 21-day program and you decide to "fall off" at the end, you can always come back to yourself with mindful awareness and continue the process of refining all the different pieces.

Many diet and health books talk about the specific foods that you need to eat to lose weight or to be healthy. Or the exercise that you have to do. But instead I want you to look at how different foods make you *feel*. How different exercises make you *feel*. I want you to remain aware of how different things impact you, some positively, some negatively. No one, not a single doctor or researcher or coach or yoga teacher, has the perfect exercise plan that works for every single person. But mindful awareness is a universal tool that allows us to pick and choose, to see what's going to be most helpful for us personally in the long term.

Is it helpful for us to eat a deprivation diet of kale juice or lemon water, or to start fasting? Is it helpful to follow really specific diets or restrict certain foods? Is it more useful to look for the things that will help us to feel better and stay on track? That's what mindfulness does: helps us to build up our health by paying attention to how we feel *after* we make our choices—so we can make better ones, if needed, next time.

Our metabolism is a reflection of our health. As

our systems begin to reset, our body's metabolism balances, resulting in a more glowing outward reflection. And mindfulness also helps us tap in to the most important part: how we feel. Our outlook is determined not merely by our physical health but also by our mental and spiritual health: *How do I see the world? How do I see myself? How do I feel in my body? How do I feel within my environment? How do I feel in my interactions with people?* How we feel impacts our reactions and choices in each of these areas, leading us either into downward spirals of disease, muscle atrophy, and more fat tissue, or into upward spirals of vital health and lean, healthy tissue.

Today, as we approach the end of your first Meditate Your Weight cycle, I want to encourage you to keep going—extend this program beyond tomorrow. If you can hold on to the commitment you've made to mindfulness, all of your weight-related concerns will naturally fall into place.

The secret, one of the most important yet hardest things to maintain, is mindfulness without judgment. Sometimes our judgments come in to cloud our vision and we end up looking through distorted lenses. What we want to do is clean off the lenses so that we can see clearly what affects us and how.

Rather than saying, *Oh, this or that is bad for me,* or *I should never eat this, but I should always do this,* really pay attention to what's right or wrong for *you.* Mindfulness will always guide you back home.

Meditation also helps us to live with moderation, so we can better enjoy ourselves without jeopardizing our progress. For health and vitality, we need to have time to enjoy our lives. That doesn't mean we have to go out and eat cake for breakfast, lunch, and dinner— but it does mean that we can spend some time having fun with our friends. Mindfulness helps us recognize the mental and spiritual benefit of letting ourselves enjoy things. It helps us manage the hardest part about moderation: the judgment we impose when we allow ourselves to do that, as well as our ability to remain aware of when enough is enough. Mindfulness helps us remember that there's a time to be outwardly focused and social, and there's a time to be inwardly focused and really pay attention to our health. We might spend our vacation whooping it up with friends, but afterward (or even at some point during), we can spend time coming back to that mindfulness in how we eat, move, and live, to recover that balance. This awareness helps us to learn to know the difference.

Today's meditation is about committing to health unfolding as a journey. Begin with the simple observation meditation that we've been doing. Now we'll focus on the awareness of health as a process of balance. Feel a sense of heaviness in the legs and the pelvis anchoring you down to the ground and the sense of stability that it creates physically and mentally. Feel the connection to the earth beneath you and the sense of strength and structure that the lower body creates.

Then notice the lightness in the upper body. Feel the head and rib cage floating lightly upward, giving the upper body a sense of flexibility and adaptability. Notice the combination of lightness and flexibility in the upper body with a balance of strength and steadiness in the lower body. Recognize your ability to create that, just with this experience in your body. This experience of those two opposites helps us to recognize that we are able to find balance and steadiness; we are able to commit to something as well as have the ability to be flexible along the way.

Mind Makeover

Today, in your journal:

1. Write about one simple change that you can commit to for the next 30 days. It can be one of the changes you committed to earlier in the program—that's totally fine. Here's some advice to help you choose: What changes have you made in the last three weeks that have been the most successful? Did mindfulness help you realize that you do better when you have more protein with breakfast? Or maybe running doesn't really agree with you, but attending two or three yoga classes per week does the trick? Or maybe you realized that you have trouble seeing yourself as anything but fat. Perhaps your 30-day commitment is going back to day 18 and repeating it for 30 days, until you can call up the image of your lean self without any difficulty whatsoever.

   One caution: Don't say something like, *I'm going to eat better for a month.* Make it clear and specific. Picking one thing to make your priority for the next 30 days allows you to make significant progress and train your brain for the most impactful change, ensuring that it will become a habit.

2. Write down your goals for the year, the next five years, ten years. Create goals for work, family, health, and other areas. These might be pie-in-the-sky goals—the important thing is to just write them down.

3. Look at your 30-day commitment again. What does that one commitment look like after a month? One year? Ten years? Does that commitment change over those periods? How will your day-to-day priorities align with the goals you've created? Where will you be spending your time based on those priorities?

....

TODAY'S MANTRA:
I am committed to feeling great.

....

Building Awareness

Notice how and where you spend your time today in relation to your 30-day commitment and your other long-range goals. Notice how you normally spend and ration your time. Remind yourself that your health is important for you and the people around you. Consider how you will help yourself commit to the process of health, making it a priority, knowing that it is a long-term, ongoing process, and not an end point.

....

*"I am here to share my
gifts with the world."*

Each of us is born with a unique skill set and character, with strengths and limitations, and each of us
is meant to contribute to this world in a unique way.
We may not be clear on what exactly that is, and it
may change over time, but we each have a unique
design. Once you recognize this truth and start living
from it, the distractions in your life will seem much
less significant. You will start to see the larger goal of
great health as an offering to the world for the gifts
you've been given.

Eating to feed your health and mental capacity,
taking time to refuel, noticing how you limit yourself
with your perspective—all of these changes will lead
to better service to our families and our communities, even the larger, global community. You can now

see your unique gifts to the world, as well as how you can be more efficient and effective when you are comfortable in your body and clear in your mind. You are recognizing that to do your best work in life, you need to be at your best.

Now our question is: How do we live up to this new and clarified image? How do we take this potential out into the world? And where do we go from here?

The final day of the program, I want you to think about how you will share yourself with the world. Over these past few weeks, you've looked at your physical health as well as reflected on how you look and feel. You've thought about feeling sexy, looking at yourself differently, loving your body. You've considered your strengths, and how those inner strengths contribute to your outer beauty. You've looked at how you share those gifts with the world, how our "flaws" connect us with the people around us.

You have taken time to consider how much you have to offer, and you have started to really shift your perspective on yourself and the world around you. Now that you can clearly see all of your gifts and your self-limiting mental patterns, I ask: How dare you not step into the world with purpose? *How dare you not live up to your potential?*

The world needs something from each of us. Our unique contribution to the world might change many times—sometimes it might be to care for our families, or to run a business, or to work for the common good, or to create art. Our duty is to step into the world with a sense of purpose, a sense of connection to our community, and our full ability to utilize our gifts.

We've talked about our outer beauty being only so deep. About how it's our strengths that really allow us to be radiant. And most important is our need to connect with and to support those around us so we can find a sense of meaning and purpose and depth in our lives.

Most of all, I want you to remind yourself why you're here. We started the book talking about how easy it is to get caught up in images in the magazines and an idea of what we should look like. And a few days ago we talked about how important it is to recognize that our imperfections are what connect us to one another and make us more well-rounded and real. Our unique strengths allow us to contribute in a way that's really meaningful to this world, and to support the people around us. And we know how important it is to accept support from the people around us as well—which helps our loved ones fulfill their purpose, too.

Mindfulness is coming back to all of these lessons, without judgment. Many of us remember growing up with a sense of parental expectations that we become a doctor or lawyer, preconceived notions of what we should be or what's a "good" job. But we know that every job has such an important purpose to this world, and that each one of us is made for different things. Once we realize that we are able to access those gifts and contribute them to the world, we start to approach our lives in a very different way. Instead of being bogged down in how many calories we eat every day, we start to live from a place of feeling good about ourselves, wanting to be healthy instead of trying to deprive ourselves to get the perfect gym body. We start to live from a place of self-worth, and of feeling good to be able to contribute something meaningful to this world.

(If 12 minutes doesn't feel comfortable for you, stay at 10.) Begin by paying attention to the natural flow of your breath. Then train your focus on the potential at your fingertips. Visualize a balance of giving and receiving—of both giving support to your communities around you, and giving your gifts to your work, family, and self, as well as receiving the support that you need from the people around you. You'll notice a sense of health and vitality in recognizing your ability to cultivate this sense of balance. As you visualize this potential at your fingertips as a balance of in and out, of giving and receiving, continue to observe your breath. Now, on the inhale, take in nourishment. On the exhale, allow the exhaled breath to be an offering. Notice how this balance keeps you nourished so you don't need to run on empty anymore. Also see how it helps to nourish the people and community around you.

Mind Makeover

In today's journaling, answer the following:

1. What is your untapped potential that you're waiting to share with the world? How has your weight and/or health held you back from using that untapped potential—until now?

2. What does the world need from you?

Serving your company, raising your children, doing volunteer work, feeding your family, whatever that is—what does the world need from you?

3. What is one positive attribute that you would like to have become part of your character? Most of us have certain things we'd like to improve upon—to be less selfish, or more punctual, or more positive. Just list one attribute.

....

TODAY'S MANTRA:
I am here to share my gifts with the world.

....

Building Awareness

Your awareness for today is about your chosen attribute. As you go through your day, be aware of moments in which you can explore and attend to this attribute. Perhaps you'd like to be braver and take more risks, so you approach a neighbor you've been wanting to befriend. Perhaps you want more energy, so you sign up for a new spinning class or you take a brisk walk at lunch. Consider how much greater your ability to key in to this attribute has grown since you began the program three weeks ago. You can even continue on this chosen attribute tomorrow, as you begin your 30-day commitment cycle.

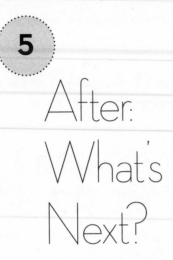

5

After: What's Next?

I hope that these past three weeks have been a gentle, simple introduction to the powerful practice of meditation. Mindful awareness can be a health-changing (and life-changing) habit. At the end of these 21 days, perhaps you've developed a meditation habit that you feel confident will remain in your life for months and years to come. If you'd like to extend your practice, you have more than a few options. Let's discuss some here.

Repeat the program: Many people feel supported and safe inside this 21-day program—but they fear being "done" because they're convinced they'll lose ground without a system to guide them and spur them on. If that sounds like you, feel free to simply repeat the 21-day program—even several times— digging a bit deeper into each day's material and extending the meditations to match your current duration for each session. (Remember when meditating for 3 minutes felt *so long*?)

Pick a day to focus on: You can also return to any day that was either difficult for you or especially helpful. As we go through these 21 days, most of us discover at least one or two days that were extremely hard to connect with—which is often a good sign of an area that could stand a bit more investigation.

Alternately, another day may have felt extraordinarily helpful to you—that would also be a good one to go back and repeat. You likely have more than one day's contemplation material there. (We all have at least one day like that!) You could repeat it once or twice, or as needed, or even for three months. Inside of each day's meditation, you can explore many aspects of each theme. You may repeat any and all of the days, as often as you like.

Return to day 18: The visualization on day 18 is one that I'd recommend coming back to, and even repeating daily for a month, especially if you've had trouble losing weight. I think this concept—that we cannot change until our brains believe it is possible—is one of the most powerful parts of the process. Meditation helps our entire nervous system go to work to create the expectations of our brain. And so if our brain expects us to be fat and it can't get around the idea of that, your nervous system and body will find it very difficult to create a different reality. My patients have found it extremely helpful to repeat that day for three weeks or even a month, meditating for 5 or 10 minutes each time. As we've discussed, a big part of any weight-loss program is not just eating the right foods and exercising but also shifting our mind-sets and increasing awareness of our expectations. I've seen elevated expectations manifest in a very real way almost immediately. As soon as we expect ourselves to be healthy, we start to eat differently. We start to choose differently. Not because we're judging ourselves or because we're "sticking to" a diet that forces our hand and tells us we have to eat a certain way— but because we're paying attention and noticing what it feels like to be our healthy selves. Our mindfulness helps us deeply appreciate this change, so we become grateful and can genuinely enjoy health. These are the kinds of changes that are ultimately sustainable because they feel so good.

Focus on your chosen attribute: Don't forget that you'll also continue with a 30-day commitment to a change you chose on day 20. You might use the following format for your meditations:

> Now is the time to be an observer. Sit and observe your breath. Trying not to change the breath, start to notice what your chosen attribute looks like. Spend some time just visualizing yourself having that quality, whether it's generosity or positivity or determination. Notice how you will go through your day differently with that quality. How you carry yourself differently. How you interact with people differently. Visualize tucking yourself in to bed at night, and notice how differently you feel at the end of the day spent embodying that one characteristic.

Once you feel comfortable with your habit and attribute, you don't need to spend your entire time meditating on it, but having this focus can help ground you at the beginning or the end of the meditation. The idea is that, as we start to pay attention to these qualities, we train ourselves to use this habit or attribute. Eventually, it becomes part of us—and shifts us away from the parts of us we don't want to grow.

Extend the length of your meditation: I always recommend that beginning meditators start small and stick with an easy length of time until they *really* feel like they want to do more. The most enduring shift is when you get to the point at which you feel like you *need* more and you can't wait to sit longer.

If you're starting to get that feeling, just add maybe 2 to 5 minutes at a time—and never add on more than 5 minutes at any one time. Remind yourself that progressing at that pace, if it proves sustainable, would be really impressive—you could have added 15 to 30 minutes to your session in just a week's time! Resist that ego drive to catapult up to the big leagues of an hour a day—chances are, your overeagerness will backfire, and your habit will be compromised. Don't let that happen! Slow, steady, and sustainable always wins.

Try meditating a different way: If you're curious about what else is out there, explore! Meditation comes in so many forms. Some people meditate with their eyes open, while staring at things. Other people chant or repeat affirmations in their mind. With as many different techniques as you will find, remember not to get too distracted by the bells and whistles—at its root, meditation is all just mindful awareness of the natural inner processes of the body and the breath. Unless you want one, you don't need to have a focal point—and you definitely don't have to do any exotic chants, breathing, or other specialized business, unless you want to.

One of the most versatile meditations is simply counting your breath:

> Just as we've done throughout the program, observe the breath, and simply count your breaths. A full cycle of a single inhalation and a single exhalation would count as 1. The next inhale and exhale would be 2. Ideally, you get to 10, then start over. But many times you'll either lose your place or end up at 20, or 15, or 25. But as soon as you remember, you just bring it back to 1.

This technique is just a great way to give the mind something to chew on for those days when your monkey mind is jumping all over the place, and you feel like just sitting down and watching the breath isn't enough.

Consistency is key: Even if all you're doing is 2 minutes of observing your breath, continuing with your daily practice is what's most important. By now, you may sense that you're beginning to use the awareness you've created, in so many areas of your life, to unlock your potential. Look at how much you've learned in this process toward health—continuing your daily mindfulness can help you delve deeper for more insights and more growth.

Above all, be gentle with yourself: Many of us end up walking through our lives on autopilot. Going through the motions—clocking in, clocking out, coming home, making dinner, kissing our kids good night. All of these are part of life, and there's no avoiding a certain amount of monotony. But very often we go through the motions of what we think our lives should be for years, and when we finally step back and get clarity on what that looks like, we can be shocked. *Oh, wow—I'm actually really unhappy.* Or even *Oh, wow—this is much better than I was thinking it was!*

Some people, when they begin meditating, experience a period of grief when they realize how much of their lives they've been missing. No matter what phase of life you're in, whether you're just out of college or in your seventies, the process of waking up can be really exhilarating and exciting, a fresh start. But it can also serve as a reminder of how much time has been lost or wasted. Yet while meditation may provide this clarity, it will not abandon you in it. What can keep you on track through this grief is saying, *Well, how do I choose now?*

Some come to these types of wellness programs seeking transformation—and they may find it. When people who haven't meditated before begin to slow down and do a regular meditation practice, they find themselves clarifying major questions in their lives and may experience big changes, such as finding fulfilling relationships (or leaving unhealthy ones) or leaping forward in their career (or shifting to a new line of work). In my experience, it would be more unusual if people *don't* experience life changes after making meditation a regular practice.

But to me, meditation is not necessarily about realizing what's broken and fixing it. Instead, it's about gaining the clarity to reveal true happiness and contentment. The critical part of starting to meditate is that you are able to wipe away your judgment of yourself. You are able to completely redefine what you think about your life or what you're capable of doing—or what you think you should be doing. Now you are able to come to these major life questions without preconceived notions and just look.

Ultimately, this program is about developing mindfulness, not only for those few minutes spent in meditation but throughout the rest of the day as well. *Mindfulness* is one of those catchwords these days—but in reality, all it means is, *I'm paying attention. I'm paying attention to my thoughts and feelings. I'm paying attention to the sugar craving and asking where it's coming from. I'm not judging the craving— I'm merely gathering data. Did I eat well this morning? Am I under negative stress? Am I nervous about a big date tonight? Maybe I should start eating more regularly. Or maybe I'm just craving sugar because I'm out with my friends and I'm having fun. Maybe I'll just eat it, enjoy it, and move on to the rest of my glorious life.*

Mindfulness flexes to fit into the full range of human experience—indeed, it helps you experience this full range. Mindfulness meditation is a discipline with a versatile set of skills that can see you through all phases of your life. Once you've internalized these skills and committed to a daily practice, you'll have mindful awareness guiding you through every trying transition, maximizing every joyful experience, helping you derive the most resonance and meaning out of every moment of your life.

Not bad for a few quiet minutes in your room, right?

THE MEDITATE YOUR WEIGHT TOOL KIT

....

Part 3

....

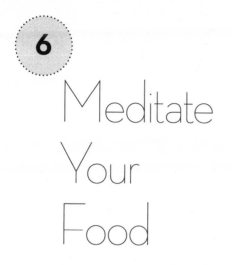

6

Meditate
Your
Food

Changing the focus from losing weight to gaining health helps in every area of our lives—especially in the way we eat. Many times we get caught in the cycle of eating as a reaction to craving, becoming reactive instead of proactive. I hope that the Meditate Your Weight program has helped get you out of that reactive mode, so you can be more deliberate and intentional about your health.

Once we begin to look at food as a form of nourishment, as opposed to a sparring partner in a lifelong love/hate relationship, we begin to choose foods that will help us optimize our functioning—and a smoothly running metabolism becomes a happy side effect. Focusing on the nutrient composition of your foods and studying your personal reactions to these foods, you will start to feel the way these fuel you differently than junk carbs or other nutritionally bankrupt foods do.

If you can make that connection, you can train yourself to crave different foods. You can eventually eat high-quality, vitality-amping foods in the same way you once ate nutritionally bankrupt ones—because they make you feel better.

The Meditate Your Weight approach works with any type of eating plan. So if you're a vegetarian, Paleo-lover, vegan, or what have you, and that eating plan suits you, please feel free to carry on. If you're feeling like you need a little more guidance, here are a few basics that can help you get the most from your food.

CREATE YOUR OWN FOOD ATLAS

Think of yourself as an explorer of your body's patterns and habits. When explorers first go into uncharted territory, they don't have a frame of reference, so they have to pick out landmarks to help them get a clearer picture of where they are. As you move through the Meditate Your Weight program, use mindfulness to note a few key "landmarks" to help you navigate toward the best plan for you. Notice your level of hunger and energy:

- between meals
- directly before and after meals
- about two hours after meals

Notice the quality of your hunger—do you often experience a growling in your stomach? Or do you find that your mind directs you to think about food according to the clock (that is, around set meal times)? Note how different foods and combinations of foods affect you. Here's an example of how you might map your eating pattern.

My current food atlas:

I notice I have a tendency to get really tired

> *at three in the afternoon. And I also have*
> *a tendency not to eat at all until noon. And*
> *then I eat a lot of carbs, which tends to set*
> *me up for a crash about an hour later.*

My revised food atlas:

> *I really need to be able to make sure that*
> *I eat something in the morning, even if I'm*
> *not hungry. And then a little bit of some-*
> *thing, maybe as a separate snack, or a bite*
> *before a meal, so as not to go into lunch*
> *starving and eat too much. That will help*
> *me sustain my energy in the afternoon.*

As you continue your food exploration, you can add details. Note your eating habits and tendencies, your energy level, how your body reacts to certain foods. As your food atlas gets filled out, you'll have a better picture of your entire experience with food.

Time	Hunger/ Energy Level Before	I Ate . . .	Hunger/ Energy Level After	Hunger/ Energy Level 2 Hours Later

PAY ATTENTION TO FOOD QUALITY: ELIMINATE THE BIG 5

Food quality is very important. You could do this entire program and reap wonderful benefits, but if you're not eating decent food and paying attention, you're missing a huge piece of the puzzle.

Most prepared or pre-packaged food is high in sugars and low in nutritional value. Consider starting your transition away from processed foods by eating very simple whole foods, so you can more easily see how individual foods make you feel. When you eat mindfully, you'll notice your cravings and what's really behind them: *I'm craving sugar. Why is that? Well, I haven't eaten for five hours. And my body is really smart. My body knows sugar is instant energy. What it doesn't know is that after that instant energy, I am going to crash. When I start to crave things like sugar, a lot of times it's that I didn't really feed myself properly. That set me up. I waited too long, or I ate foods that didn't carry me through.*

So what will carry you through? That will depend on what works best in your unique body. But one of the easiest ways to radically and immediately improve the quality of your food is to eliminate what

I call the Big 5: sugar, wheat, dairy, alcohol, and caffeine.

1. **Sugar:** Sugar overconsumption wreaks havoc with our immune and endocrine systems, leading to chronic conditions such as arthritis, osteoporosis, diabetes, asthma, and hypoglycemia, as well as cavities and periodontal disease. One of the best ways to support your immune system, protect your digestion and cellular health, normalize your blood sugar and metabolism, and lose weight is to decrease the amount of sugar in your diet. On average, each American consumes more than 150 pounds of sugar and related sweeteners per year. There are obvious sources—such as the seventeen teaspoons in each can of cola—but there are also many hidden ones in the common foods we eat. Here are some hidden (and not-so-hidden) sources of sugar:

   • salad dressings
   • sauces (most restaurants not only use

unhealthy oils and salt but usually add plenty of sugar as well)

- condiments (ketchup, pickles, mustard, jelly, mayonnaise)
- breads and pastries
- rice, soy, and nut milks
- juices, Gatorade, coffee drinks
- most prepared/packaged food (snacks, frozen entrées, canned soup, packaged cereal, frozen waffles, crackers)

This last one is a killer: The common combination of sugar and grains in processed foods stimulates the pancreas to release a tremendous amount of insulin—so much that our cells can eventually become resistant to it, and insulin resistance is a stepping-stone to diabetes.

Try to cut out all refined sweeteners—especially white sugar and high-fructose corn syrup—and to limit natural sweeteners, such as honey, maple syrup, or agave, as much as possible. But be aware that when we stop eating high-sugar foods, our body takes several days to lower our insulin levels. In the meantime, the high insulin levels can prompt symptoms such as dizziness, confusion, headaches, and generally feeling miserable. While you're transitioning off high-sugar foods, try to eat some protein and/or fiber every two hours for the first few days, to help stabilize your blood sugar.

2. **Wheat:** Most Americans consume an enormous amount of wheat on a daily basis, which is why wheat is one of the most commonly acquired food sensitivities (along with dairy, corn, and soy). Wheat can inhibit the normal functioning of your thyroid, which can lead to a slowdown in metabolism. Overconsumption of wheat products causes your blood sugar to spike and can also lead to systemic inflammation and leaky gut syndrome, both of which have implications for body weight.

   If you have thyroid issues, digestive problems, or difficulty losing weight, try cutting wheat out completely for a couple of weeks and see how you feel. If you feel better in any significant way (more energy, easier digestion, less intense allergies, or smoother skin, for example), removing wheat may be an important step in revitalizing your metabolism. If this is the case, it may be best to cut wheat out of your diet for the long term.

If you do this test and don't experience any obvious changes, try to limit wheat to just once or twice a week, and use this measure as a way of cultivating more variety in what you eat. Substitute nutritious grains, such as amaranth, quinoa, faro, millet, oats, buckwheat, and brown/basmati rice, to give your diet a more diverse nutrient profile. The wider the variety of nutrients you ingest, the healthier, more satisfied, and more nourished your body will feel.

3. **Dairy:** In Chinese medicine, dairy is considered a mucus-forming food that, in excess, can slow down your metabolic engine. Lactose intolerance is a common

cause of bloating and intestinal upset, affecting one out of five Caucasians and four out of five Asians and Native Americans. Some people find it extremely difficult to cut dairy (especially cheese) out of their diet—which may be related to milk's casein, a protein that has opioid effects in the brain. While research on dairy's impact on weight loss is mixed, many find that they simply feel lighter and cleaner when they kick dairy.

This may be a hard rule to swallow, especially for women who were raised with the "Got milk?" slogan and have considered dairy their main source of the calcium believed to strengthen bones and thus help prevent osteoporosis and other diseases. However, many other foods have highly bioavailable sources of calcium, such as dark green leafy vegetables (kale, chard, and collard greens), nuts, seeds, and whole grains.

We're lucky to live in a time with many dairy substitutes and more being developed every day. (Thank you, vegan chefs!) Have fun exploring the many va-

rieties of nondairy milks—such as coconut, almond, and cashew—as well as
yogurts and cheeses. And don't forget
about other foods with similar creamy
textures, such as avocado, which you can
use as a thickener in your smoothies or
other recipes.

4. **Alcohol:** Have you ever heard the saying
"Don't drink your calories"? Well, alcohol
is extremely high in sugar and calories—
but that's just the start of its effect on
weight and health. We all know that alcohol loosens our inhibitions, which can
make sticking to a program very difficult. But alcohol also interferes with the
function of the liver, the most important
organ for cleaning toxins from the body.
Alcohol elevates stress hormones and
disrupts sleep cycles, making sleep less
deep and restorative and keeping blood
sugar elevated overnight. Alcohol also in-
teracts with GABA receptors and blocks
the brain's oxygen sensors, complicating
sleep conditions like sleep apnea (which
has also been linked to obesity).

Now, I'm not saying to never drink again. Go ahead and enjoy a glass of wine or two, in moderation, a couple of nights a week, if you like it. But even with the widely hailed antioxidant benefits of red wine, I still recommend keeping four to five days of your week alcohol-free to allow the liver to rest so it can properly metabolize your food and detoxify the body.

5. **Caffeine:** Caffeine is the great pretender—it masks our true energy levels and hinders our ability to tune in to what our body really needs. In a mindful approach to health, that masking effect is probably the most important thing to consider when looking at your relationship to caffeine.

Caffeine is a powerful stimulant; even in small doses it blocks neurotransmitters for sleep and throws off the body's natural circadian rhythm. Caffeine also excites the adrenals, the glands that regulate stress, which are already overused and overstimulated due to our hectic lifestyles. Caffeine keeps already high cortisol levels chronically elevated, thereby helping to pack on extra belly fat.

Our favorite source of caffeine is coffee. Coffee interferes with your cells' ability to use water. It also quickly depletes the calcium and magnesium stores your body needs for bone health, muscle contraction, and relaxation. Without those stores, your body is less able to release spasms and to allow your muscles to stretch more like elastic and less like a wire. And even with all the recent news of coffee's positive effects, the jury is still out on how it affects cholesterol, insulin control, blood vessels, rheumatoid arthritis, and more.

Perhaps even more important to consider: Coffee beans are frequently grown in countries where regulations on pesticide use are less restrictive than in the United States. If you do drink coffee, drink organically grown beans to protect the health of the people working in the coffee fields and minimize their toxic exposure to the pesticides as well as your own.

OBSERVE A FEW SIMPLE EATING RULES

Our bodies respond differently to different kinds of foods. I'm not here to prescribe a certain diet—you can decide that for yourself (hopefully with the use of mindful attention and your food atlas). Here are a few rules that I've found most useful with my clients. (I've adapted a few of these from my first book, *Optimal Health for a Vibrant Life*.)

1. Eat slowly, chew your food thoroughly, and enjoy the act of nourishing yourself. Just thinking about food causes you to salivate and release enzymes in your stomach, which is the start of the healthy digestive process. Eating slowly helps your body take full advantage of all steps of healthy digestion—including how it helps you realize when you're full.

2. Stop eating when you are 75 percent full. Give your food time to hit your stomach. If you are still hungry 30 minutes later, eat some more.

3. Try not to go longer than 3 to 4 hours between meals.

4. Do not eat standing up, at your computer, or watching television. Sit, enjoy, relax, and chew!

5. Do not eat after 8 p.m.

6. If you find yourself craving carbohydrates and sugar, have a snack with mostly protein or fat, then wait 30 minutes. Protein and fat are more satisfying than carbs and sugar, and they are usually what your body is really craving. Fats trigger the satiety response, making you feel fuller.

7. Throw away your scale. Measure your success by how you feel.

8. Don't count calories. Go by how clean and nourishing your food is. Eat what you like, but use moderation and variety. Most of all, get creative!

9. Usually the hardest part of balanced eating is making sure you get enough protein and vegetables. Cook enough food at each meal so that you always have leftovers on hand to eat later or mix in with other nutritious foods.

10. Limit your fluid intake with meals, as it

dilutes gastric enzymes, making it more difficult to digest the food. A small glass of room-temperature water with your meal is plenty.

THE MEDITATE YOUR WEIGHT APPROACH TO MEALS

BREAKFAST

Eat breakfast with protein; cereal and muffins hurt more than help. Protein starts the metabolic fire early in the day; otherwise your body starts hoarding and enters starvation mode. Breakfast supplies the nutrients for your day, so choose mindfully. A protein-rich smoothie is a great way to start.

LUNCH

Make a sandwich that's heavy on the insides; in other words, the inner part of the sandwich outweighs the bread part. Start with whole grain bread. Pile on plenty of veggies: lettuce, tomato, onions. Here's a good place to use leftover steamed veggies cooked the night before. Add some freshly cooked or leftover nitrate-free meat. Slather on a spread to add some good fats that will stabilize the blood sugar: organic butter, avocado, pesto, hummus, or whatever you like to add a little flavor and moisture. Watch out for bad oils (especially partially-hydrogenated or palm oils) and added preservatives and sugars in whatever you're spreading. Put it all together and slice the sandwich in half. Eat the whole thing, or eat half at lunch and the other half 2 to 4 hours later. A sandwich is easy to take with you, too. If you can't pack your lunch, or you're not a sammy fan, order a salad with some protein in it.

In the winter I like to make a big pot of soup at the beginning of the week. I make it very simple— broth and veggies and some protein—and then I add to it for different meals. In the spring and summer, I buy lots of fresh veggies so my fridge is like a giant salad bar. The key is to eat small portions often, using whole foods as much as possible.

DINNER

Keep it simple. Pick some veggies and steam or stir-fry them. Use coconut oil or butter when making a stir-fry, as these won't hydrogenate like other fats when cooking at higher temperatures. After the veggies are cooked, add a little olive oil and sea salt—unrefined sea salt should be pink or grayish. I like this combination with lightly cooked veggies because I can taste the subtleties of the food. You can also try lemon, honey, and olive oil mixed with salt. Spices are good, too. Once you get the hang of it you can play with sauces.

Then pick a meat or meat substitute: fish, chicken, lamb, beef, beans, tofu, tempeh, a combination. Steam, bake, barbecue, or stir-fry. Olive oil and sea salt are great flavorings for meat, too.

If you have time, add a whole-grain dish such as quinoa, brown rice, millet, or amaranth. Quinoa contains lots of protein and minerals and is quick and easy, taking only 15 minutes to cook once it boils. If you're unsure how to cook any of these grains, you can usually find both great recipes and instructions online. A rice cooker/steamer is very handy.

If you want something sweet, eat a piece of fruit an hour or two after dinner or chop up some fruit to make a fruit salad and mix it with unsweetened, organic coconut yogurt.

Above all, enjoy!

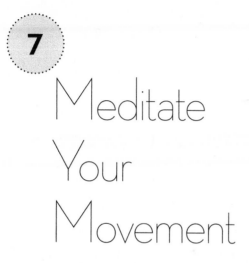

Meditate
Your
Movement

When I counsel my patients about exercise in relation to losing weight, I repeatedly stress one point:
The most important thing is to find an activity that
you love to do, and do that. Full stop, the end. You
need almost no other rules.

If you don't like running, don't run. If you don't
like to go to the gym, don't go to the gym! Instead,

keep looking until you find the right fit for you, whether that is open-water swims at the local lake or Zumba in the church basement or early-morning hikes on the mountain with your dog. The enjoyment factor is essential, not only for psychological reasons. If you exercise while you're feeling tense and bitter, your body will perceive that movement differently and hold you back. Forcing yourself to do dreaded activities, gripping and tightening your shoulders and neck the whole way, will impact your muscle patterning, your nervous system response, and even your metabolism. You will never get the same benefit from exercise you resent as you do from exercise that frees you to enjoy and release yourself to the experience.

Some people's systems will function much better with 20 to 30 minutes of exercise; others will feel better with 2 hours. Some people can only manage 10 minutes a day. Any time that fits into your life and feels best to you is absolutely fine. And as with meditation, a little bit every day is preferable to a lot once a week.

Finding your exercise sweet spot may take some experimenting, but I would just love us all to get rid of the "I have to beat myself up in order to lose weight" mind-set. If you're busy and stressed, and you place expectations such as *I must work out for two hours, or it's not worth it!* on top of that, you are actively adding stress to your life and shooting yourself in the metabolic foot. Take the time to figure out what types of movement can be enjoyable and easily fit with the rhythms of your life. Your metabolism and mental health will thank you.

Because yoga can be a good supplemental practice to meditation, I've created a gentle 20-minute yoga sequence you can do to complement your meditation retreat. This practice is meant to help balance and stimulate the metabolism and the nervous system. If you're doing yoga with the meditation, it's probably best to do the yoga first, as it will open up the hips and help you sit in meditation more comfortably. If not, just know this is an optional add-on, and please continue your search for the joyful exercise that's right for you.

THE MEDITATE YOUR WEIGHT DAILY YOGA SEQUENCE

This simple sequence—a series of eight active poses and two more restorative poses—helps stimulate the circulation, restore the parasympathetic nervous system, and rev up the cardiovascular system. You can either do all ten poses in a sequence together, or you can do the two restorative poses whenever you need to downshift a bit (such as after work, before bed, or when you're feeling stressed). For the first eight poses, start with holding them 30 seconds each, and work up to holding for a full minute on each side. For the final two poses, hold them as long as feels comfortable and practical for your schedule.

Before you start, consider reading through all the instructions first, to get a sense of how much space is required (and what would be the best place in your house to practice) and any props you might need (such as a yoga mat, strap, towel, and blanket), and to generally get comfortable with the idea of the poses. You might also find it helpful to time your poses at first.

The first few times through the sequence, you might feel awkward setting up and transitioning between the poses. But, with a bit of practice, you'll be able to turn this sequence into a nice flow.

The Meditate Your Weight
Daily Yoga Sequence

The whole sequence, at a glance:

1. Cat/Cow
2. Down Dog Walking
3. Crescent
4. Down Dog Walking
5. Warrior II
6. Down Dog Walking
7. Plank Walking (Plank to Forearm Plank)
8. Bridge Pose
9. Supine Leg and Hip Stretch
10. Legs Up the Wall

1 Cat/Cow

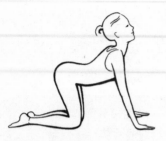

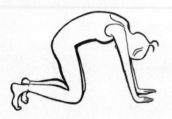

Start on your hands and knees with your hands under your shoulders and your knees under your hips. On your inhale, arch your back and drop your belly toward the floor, lifting your chest up toward the sky as you look up.

As you exhale, start to curl the belly back and up toward your spine, pushing away from the floor and tucking the chin. The spine will round and your head will drop.

Inhale again, extending the chest to look up.

Keep repeating the inhale and exhale of this pose for 30 seconds, working up to 60 seconds. Transition directly to pose 2.

2 Down Dog Walking

From pose 1, tuck your toes under, straighten your arms, and push up into Downward-Facing Dog position, straightening your legs as much as possible. Aim for a 90-degree angle in your hips. Keep your hands shoulder width apart and your feet about hip width apart. (If your hamstrings are tight, you can bend your knees a little. Eventually, the legs will be straight and the back and pelvis will be fairly flat and neutral, without rounding.)

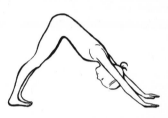

On your inhale, lift your right leg up as high as is comfortable while keeping your hips squared. On your exhale, lower it down. On your next inhale, lift your left leg; on the exhale, lower it down. Repeat for 30 seconds, building up to 60 seconds. This pose should feel like you are walking while in Downward-Facing Dog; your arms, shoulders, and back should stay in the same position throughout the exercise.

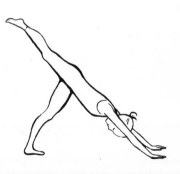

3 Crescent

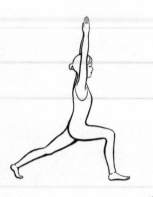

From Down Dog Walking, step your feet forward and slowly return to standing position. Then step your right leg forward and leave your left leg behind you. You'll be on the ball of the left foot, making sure that your bent right knee is aligning over the right ankle. On your inhale, take your arms up overhead, keeping the back nice and straight.

On the exhale, come halfway forward so your belly comes toward your thigh but does not actually touch it. Then, on the inhale, come back up.

Note: What you really want to feel here is your glutes and hips engaging to help steady you in the pose. Your larger, more powerful muscles in the glutes and the thighs really have to work and actively support you as you move. Also, your core will remain engaged, supporting you as you move and maintain a straight and flat spine.

Stay with the breath, moving forward and back in sync with your inhales and exhales, your legs remaining rooted and your legs holding their position. Start with 30 seconds, building up to 60 seconds. Then repeat on the left side.

After you've repeated these steps on your right and left side, step back into Downward-Facing Dog.

4 Down Dog Walking (Repeat)

Follow instructions for pose 2.

5 Warrior II

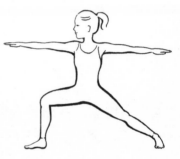

From Down Dog Walking, step your feet forward and slowly return to standing position. Then step your right foot forward about four feet from the left, with the right knee bent and aligned over the right ankle so that your kneecap is pointing forward with your right foot. Turn the back foot in about 45 degrees. Then twist your pelvis and torso toward the left side of your mat, keeping your right knee pointed forward. Extend your arms out to the sides, relax the back and shoulders, and breathe deeply. Stay here for 30 seconds, building up to 60 seconds, and then repeat on the other side.

6 Down Dog Walking (Repeat)

From Warrior II, step back into Downward-Facing Dog and repeat pose 2's instructions.

7 Plank Walking (Plank to Forearm Plank)

From Downward Dog, shift your weight forward until your shoulders are aligned above your wrists, keeping your feet hip width apart. Try to keep a neutral spine with a flat back. Use your core to help stabilize you; think about drawing the front of your ribs toward your back.

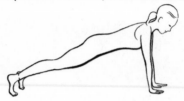

Now move into what I call Plank Walking. Lower your right forearm to the ground and pause there.

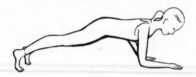

Lower your left forearm to the ground. Then raise yourself up again, taking the right hand back to the floor and straightening the right arm, then taking the left hand back to the floor and straightening the left arm. You're moving from Plank to Forearm Plank, keeping the core supported so the back stays straight. Repeat for 30 seconds and build up to a minute.

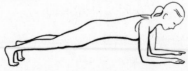

8 Bridge Pose

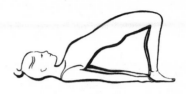

Roll your body over to transition from Plank Walking to Bridge Pose. Lie on your back with your feet on the floor about hip width apart. Lay your arms on the floor, palms down, alongside your hips. On your inhale, lift the pelvis up into the air, as high as you comfortably can. Attempt to relax your glutes, instead of clenching and gripping. Hold for 30 to 60 seconds, relaxing and breathing deeply. Exhale as you lower the pelvis.

9 Supine Leg and Hip Stretch

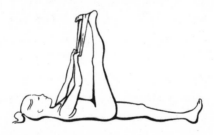

Now we transition to the restorative poses. You can also do just these last two poses during periods of high stress or in preparation for sleep.

Lie on your back, and grab a strap, towel, or sweatshirt—anything you have at hand—to loop around your legs.

Bend the right knee into the chest, and loop your strap or towel around the ball of the right foot. Slowly extend the leg straight out. You want to straighten the leg into a gentle stretch of the hamstring, only as much as you can while still relaxing the lower back, head, and pelvis on the floor. If you need to bend the knee a little bit to allow that, or take a little more slack on the strap, no problem. Hold for 30 to 60 seconds.

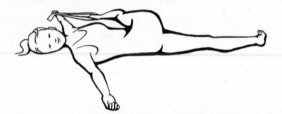

Take both ends of the strap in the left hand, and take the right leg over to the left, so your body is in a twist. Find a comfortable position where you can keep the left leg on the ground, bending the knee if necessary. You may wish to put some pillows under the legs so you can support yourself as you rest here. You want to be really comfortable in this pose as you hold for 30 to 60 seconds.

You should feel the stretch either in the outer thigh or hip or through the spine, or even in your shoulders and chest. The key to getting the most out of this whole-body stretch is to be able to relax into it, not force it.

Repeat both stretches with the left leg.

10 Legs Up the Wall

This pose is probably the most helpful for an overtaxed nervous system or reducing any trouble with sleep. To prepare, find a clear spot on a wall in your house, and have a towel or blanket nearby that's been folded to a thickness of about 2 to 3 inches. The easiest way to come into Legs Up the Wall is to lie down on your back and scoot your bottom toward the wall until you're very close. Then bend your knees and place your feet on the wall so you can lift your hips and place the blanket underneath your pelvis only. (You

want your low back to be able to relax and drape off the roll. If the height is too dramatic, refold the blanket or towel to a 1- to 2-inch thickness.) Extend your legs up the wall, lying your head back on the floor, and spread your arms out to the sides. If you have an eye pillow, now is a great time to drape it over your eyes so you can really relax. This pose helps 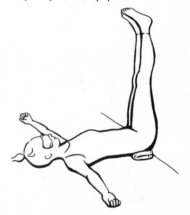 to utilize the beneficial effects of inversion on the circulation and cardiac output, allowing the blood to flow back to the heart and act as a stimulant to the circulatory system and the metabolism. For maximum benefit, try to allow yourself 3 to 5 minutes (or longer) to relax in Legs Up the Wall.

Acknowledgments

First and foremost, I want to thank the man who has supported me so much and believed in me more than anyone—the most kind and caring man I know: Forrest Hobbs.

As a kid, I was badly teased at school. Because of this experience, I continued to question myself and my worth into my adulthood. It took me many years to reassess this belief and to clearly see my value in this world. We all struggle with understanding our value, and some of this questioning never goes away. But over the past two decades of practicing yoga and meditation, I have seen that we *can* create a new relationship with our bodies and ourselves. Forrest, especially, encouraged me to be myself in the times when

I wanted to be someone else, whether I was sinking into self-doubt, or overwhelmed with work, or struggling with my own body image. He taught me the meaning of unconditional love and kindness and the joy of real partnership with someone who loves me as I am. His unwavering integrity and selfless love have inspired me in so many ways and made me more clear in my value and purpose on this planet. Without his support this book wouldn't have been possible.

I also want to thank my sister, who has been a role model to me through my struggles for so many years (especially as a teenager). Her bravery in the face of extreme obstacles inspires me in so many ways. She is the most courageous and kind woman I know.

I want to thank my parents, for blessing me with life and for their support through so many ups and downs.

And of course, I want to thank the many, many people who have made this book possible: Mariska, for bringing my ideas to life—I don't know where I would be without your help. Ashley and Tanya, for delivering my ideas to the world—without you, they would still be trapped in my head. Every yoga and meditation teacher out there, young and old, fresh-faced beginners and seasoned yogis alike, for all that you give to your communities—I am constantly inspired by you. And the many others who have supported me and loved me and urged me to write this book—it takes a tribe. Most of all, thanks to Heather Jackson and Penguin Random House for the inspiration and the push to make this happen. I am grateful to you all.

To every person out there who struggles with self-worth and feeling good in your body, I thank you for inspiring me to get this information out there. I see this book as an invitation to you to know that vibrant health is indeed possible. I hope it allows you to see the incredible potential of the mind to create and shift both your perspective and very real and tangible aspects of your physical health. If this book changes the life of just one person out there, it will have been worth the effort—and I hope it will do that for many, many more.

Endnotes

INTRODUCTION

1 Carla K. Miller et al., "Comparison of a Mindful Eating Intervention to a Diabetes Self-Management Intervention Among Adults with Type 2 Diabetes: A Randomized Controlled Trial," *Health Education and Behavior* 41, no. 2 (April 2014): 145–54, doi:10.1177/1090198113493092.

2 Hugo J. Alberts et al., "Coping with Food Cravings: Investigating the Potential of a Mindfulness-Based Intervention," *Appetite* 55, no. 1 (August 2010): 160–63, doi:10.1016.

3 Shawn N. Katterman et al., "Mindfulness Meditation as an Intervention for Binge Eating, Emotional Eating,

and Weight Loss: A Systematic Review," *Eating Behaviors* 15, no. 2 (April 2014): 197–204. doi:10.1016.

4 Jennifer Daubenmier et al., "Mindfulness Intervention for Stress Eating to Reduce Cortisol and Abdominal Fat Among Overweight and Obese Women: An Exploratory Randomized Controlled Study," *Journal of Obesity* 2011 (2011): 651936, doi:10.1155/2011/651936.

5 Eirini Christaki et al., "Stress Management Can Facilitate Weight Loss in Greek Overweight and Obese Women: A Pilot Study," *Journal of Human Nutrition and Dietetics* 26, 2 (July 2013): Supplement 132–39, doi:10.1111/jhn.12086.

CHAPTER 1: MEDITATION: THE MASTER HABIT

1 G. A. O'Reilly et al., "Mindfulness-Based Interventions for Obesity-Related Eating Behaviours: A Literature Review," *Obesity Reviews* 15, no. 6 (June 2014): 453–61, doi:10.1111/obr.12156.

2 Kavita Prasad et al., "Effect of a Single-Session Meditation Training to Reduce Stress and Improve Quality of Life Among Health Care Professionals: A 'Dose-Ranging' Feasibility Study," *Alternative Therapies in Health & Medicine* 17, no. 3 (May–June 2011): 46–49, PubMed PMID: 22164812.

3 James D. Lane, Jon Seskevich, and Carl Pieper, "Brief Meditation Training Can Improve Perceived Stress and Negative Mood," *Alternative Therapies in Health & Medicine* 13, no. 1 (January–February 2001): 38–44, PubMed PMID: 17283740.

4 Marc Wittmann et al., "Subjective Expansion of Extended Time-Spans in Experienced Meditators," *Frontiers in Psychology* 5 (January 14, 2015): 1586, doi:10.3389/fpsyg.2014.01586.

5 LONI: Laboratory of Neuro Imaging, www.loni.usc .edu/about_loni/education/brain_trivia.php.

6 Matthew A. Killingsworth and Daniel T. Gilbert, "A Wandering Mind Is an Unhappy Mind," *Science* 330, no. 6006 (November 2010): 932.

CHAPTER 2: BUSTING THROUGH YOUR MENTAL BLOCKS

1 Carla K. Miller et al., "Comparison of a Mindful Eating Intervention to a Diabetes Self-Management Intervention Among Adults with Type 2 Diabetes: A Randomized Controlled Trial," *Health Education and Behavior* 41, no. 2 (April 2014): 145–54, doi:10.1177/1090198113493092.

2 Ibid.

3 Ibid.

4 Do-Hyung Kang et al., "The Effect of Meditation on Brain Structure: Cortical Thickness Mapping and Diffusion Tensor Imaging," *Social Cognitive and Affective Neuroscience* 8, no. 1 (January 2013): 27–33, doi:10.1093/scan/nss056.

5 Jean L. Kristeller and Ruth Q. Wolever, "Mindfulness-Based Eating Awareness Training for Treating Binge Eating Disorder: The Conceptual Foundation," *Eating Disorders* 19, no. 1 (January 2011): 49–61.

6 Jean L. Kristeller and C. B. Hallett, "An Exploratory

Study of a Meditation-Based Intervention for Binge Eating Disorder," *Journal of Health Psychology* 4, no. 3 (May 1999): 357–63.

7 Kristeller and Wolever, "Mindfulness-Based Eating Awareness."

8 Ibid.

9 Miller et al., "Mindful Eating Intervention."

10 Kristeller and Wolever, "Mindfulness-Based Eating Awareness."

CHAPTER 3: MIND OVER METABOLISM

1 Jennifer Daubenmier et al., "Mindfulness Intervention for Stress Eating to Reduce Cortisol and Abdominal Fat Among Overweight and Obese Women: An Exploratory Randomized Controlled Study," *Journal of Obesity* 2011 (2011):651936, doi:10.1155/2011/651936.

2 Ashley E. Mason et al., "Acute Responses to Opioidergic Blockade as a Biomarker of Hedonic Eating Among Obese Women Enrolled in a Mindfulness-Based Weight Loss Intervention Trial," *Appetite* 91 (August 2015): 311–20.

3 Dante Cicchetti, "Resilience Under Conditions of Extreme Stress: A Multilevel Perspective," *World Psychiatry* 9, no. 3 (2010): 145–54.

4 Christine A. Maglione-Garves, Len Kravitz, and Suzanne Schneider, "Cortisol Connection: Tips on Managing Stress and Weight," Len Kravitz, Exercise Science at University of New Mexico, University of

New Mexico, www.unm.edu/~lkravitz/Article%20folder/stresscortisol.html.

5 Abiola Keller et al., "Does the Perception That Stress Affects Health Matter? The Association with Health and Mortality," *Health Psychology* 31, no. 5 (September 2012): 677–84.

6 Britta K. Hölzel et al., "Stress Reduction Correlates with Structural Changes in the Amygdala," *Social Cognitive and Affective Neuroscience* 5, no. 1 (2010): 11–17, doi:10.1093/scan/nsp034.

7 Jerath Navinder, Vernon A. Barnes, and Molly W. Crawford, "Mind-Body Response and Neurophysiological Changes During Stress and Meditation: Central Role of Homeostasis," *Journal of Biological Regulators and Homeostatic Agents* 28, no. 4 (October 2014): 545–54.

8 Ravindra Nagendra, Nirmala Maruthai, and Bindu Kutty, "Meditation and Its Regulatory Role on Sleep," *Frontiers in Neurology* 3 (April 2012): 54.

9 "Think Yourself Well," *Economist,* December 8, 2012, www.economist.com/news/science-and-technology/21567876-you-can-it-helps-think-well-yourself-first-place-think-yourself.

10 Bethany Kok et al., "How Positive Emotions Build Physical Health: Perceived Positive Social Connections Account for the Upward Spiral Between Positive Emotions and Vagal Tone," *Psychological Science* 24, no. 7 (July 1, 2013): 1123–32.

11 Nagendra, Maruthai, and Kutty, "Meditation and Its Regulatory Role."

12 Hans C. Lou et al., "A 15O-H2O PET Study of Meditation and the Resting State of Normal Consciousness," *Human Brain Mapping* 7, no. 2 (1997): 98–105.

13 Elissa Epel et al., "Can Meditation Slow Rate of Cellular Aging? Cognitive Stress, Mindfulness, and Telomeres," *Annals of the New York Academy of Sciences* 1172 (August 2009): 34–53, doi:10.1111/j.1749-6632.2009.04414.x.

14 Ergün Sahin et al., "Telomere Dysfunction Induces Metabolic and Mitochondrial Compromise," *Nature* 470, no. 7334 (February 17, 2011): 359–65, doi:10.1038/nature09787.

15 Bret Stetka, "Changing Our DNA Through Mind Control? A Study Finds Meditating Cancer Patients Are Able to Affect the Makeup of Their DNA," *Scientific American,* December 16, 2013, www.scientific american.com/article/changing-our-dna-through-mind-control/; and Linda Carlson, "Mindfulness-Based Cancer Recovery and Supportive-Expressive Therapy Maintain Telomere Length Relative to Controls in Distressed Breast Cancer Survivors," *Cancer* 121, no. 3 (February 2015): 476–84.

16 Nicola S. Schutte and John M. Malouff, "A Meta-Analytic Review of the Effects of Mindfulness Meditation on Telomerase Activity," *Psychoneuroendocrinology* 42 (April 2014): 45–48, doi:10.1016/j.psyneuen.2013.12.017.

17 Perla Kaliman et al., "Rapid Changes in Histone Deacetylases and Inflammatory Gene Expression in Expert Meditators," *Psychoneuroendocrinology* 40 (February 2014): 96–107.

18 G. A. O'Reilly et al., "Mindfulness-Based Interventions for Obesity-Related Eating Behaviors: A Literature Review," *Obesity Reviews* 15, no. 6 (2014): 453–61.

19 Rick Hanson, "Confidence: An Interview with Paul Gilbert," *The Foundation of Well-Being,* https://fwb .rickhanson.net/paul-gilbert-interviewclip.

CHAPTER 4: ESTABLISHING YOUR DAILY PRACTICE

1 Robert A. Emmons and Michael E. McCullough, "Counting Blessings Versus Burdens: An Experimental Investigation of Gratitude and Subjective Well-Being in Daily Life," *Journal of Personality and Social Psychology* 84, no. 2 (February 2003): 377–89.

2 Evon Mankarious and Emily Kothe, "A Meta-Analysis of the Effects of Measuring Theory of Planned Behaviour Constructs on Behaviour Within Prospective Studies," *Health Psychology Review* 9, no. 2 (June 2015): 190–204.

3 Jennifer R. Tomasone, Natasha Meikle, and Steven R. Bray, "Intentions and Trait Self-Control Predict Fruit and Vegetable Consumption During the Transition to First-Year University," *Journal of American College Health* 63, no. 3 (2015): 172–79.

Index

ABOUT THE AUTHOR

Internationally acclaimed yoga teacher, author, and health and wellness expert Tiffany Cruikshank is the founder of Yoga Medicine (www.YogaMedicine.com), a community of expert yoga teachers focused on fusing the best of anatomy and Western medicine with the traditional practice of yoga. Known as a "teacher's teacher," Tiffany has a master's degree in acupuncture and Oriental medicine with a specialization in sports medicine and orthopedics. In her decades of private practice and more than six years as the acupuncturist and yoga teacher at the Nike World Headquarters in Portland, Oregon, Tiffany has worked with professional athletes and performing artists from around the world. She has treated more than 25,000 patients using yoga, acupuncture, nutrition, and holistic health, collaborating with diverse health care practitioners from all disciplines to provide the best possible integrated care to her patients. Tiffany has been featured in *Yoga Journal, Prevention, Forbes,* the *Wall Street Journal, Self, Marie Claire, Fitness, Good Housekeeping, Cosmopolitan, Redbook, Mantra, Thrive, More, OM Yoga, YogaLife,* and on Fox News, among many others.